THE LITTLE BOOK OF

Mum Hacks

THE LITTLE BOOK OF

Mum Hacks

KATE MURNANE

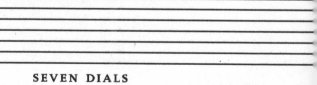

SEVEN DIALS

First published in Great Britain in 2021 by Seven Dials
an imprint of The Orion Publishing Group Ltd
Carmelite House, 50 Victoria Embankment
London EC4Y 0DZ

An Hachette UK Company

1 3 5 7 9 10 8 6 4 2

Text © Kate Murnane Limited 2021
Illustrations by Emanuel Santos
Images on pp.80-1, 128-9, 146 and 244-5 Shutterstock

A CIP catalogue record for this book is available
from the British Library.

ISBN (Hardback) 9781841884684
ISBN (eBook) 9781841884691

Printed and bound in Great Britain by Clays Ltd, Elcograf S.p.A.

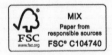

www.orionbooks.co.uk

Contents

Introduction

Hello,

This feels rather strange. I'm used to introducing myself in video form and not on the pages of a book but, nonetheless, I would still very much like to welcome you! My name's Kate and I'm a mum to two little boys, Archie and Elliot. For the last ten years I've been creating videos on YouTube. It started as a place to share my love of fashion and beauty in my early twenties but, as the years went on and my life changed, I found that my audience was growing with me and going through many of the same life stages as I was – one of those being becoming a mum.

I loved sharing my journey and the things I learnt along the way. Everything from how I was feeling in the first trimester of pregnancy to what I was packing in my hospital bag. Becoming a mum has been by far the most incredible, emotional, terrifying, wonderful life-changing journey of my life, which I think is the case for most of us. If you're a new mum-to-be, you've got all of this to look forward to!

I still remember so vividly that first night in the hospital with my new baby; I hadn't so much as changed a nappy in my life and suddenly I was expected to keep a tiny baby alive! I actually learnt my first ever mum hack that very night, (I won't ruin it for you but 'The Vest Hack' which you'll find under Newborn Hacks came in handy straight away!)

I don't profess to be a 'Super Mum' or to know everything, but I have tried and tested many hacks, tips and tricks over the years in the hope of making life a little bit easier and I feel so honoured to be able to share them with you all in one place, in this little book. Whether you're sitting reading this with a baby wriggling in your belly, hoping to gain some tips to get ahead of the game, or you're already rushing around after a little one with only five minutes to spare here and there, I wanted to make this book really easy for you to use. So, feel free to dip in and dip out for different stages and just pick this book up when you can and read only the pages that are relevant to you. This is a book for *you*, so don't feel any pressure to read it cover to cover. However you choose to read this little book, I hope you will find something to try that will make your day run that bit more smoothly or something you can incorporate into your routine.

While becoming a mum has been without question the best thing that's ever happened to me, nothing this good comes easy and some days are filled with guilt or self-doubt. It can be tempting to look at others' social media highlights and happy snapshots and assume they're an accurate and full depiction of their lives but really, deep down, we all have the same worries and fears which boil down to: Am I a good enough mum? If you're even asking yourself this question then the answer is, most probably, hell yes! So, before we get started, if you take one thing away from this book (although I hope you will take away many great tips and ideas) it's that Perfect Mums don't exist. All we can do is try our best, and if there's a way to do something quicker or more efficiently to enable us to free up more of that one thing we can't get enough of (time!) then that's something to celebrate. And of course, even though this book has come from the mind of a mum, and so is called *The Little Book of Mum Hacks*, it's also the perfect survival guide for dads too!

I would be absolutely thrilled to see you with your book so please tag me, @katebowbow, in your pictures on Instagram with #TheLittleBookofMumHacks

Kate x

Pregnancy Hacks

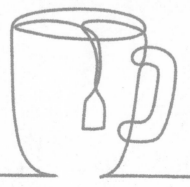

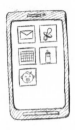

From the moment you see those two lines slowly start to appear, or the word 'pregnant' flash up on a pregnancy test, your whole world changes. I remember so clearly finding out that I was pregnant with my first son, Archie. I wasn't really feeling many symptoms, but my period was late and I had a test at home, so one evening, just after Rikki, my husband, had left for football training, I took the test. Even though I so desperately wanted a baby, nothing could prepare me for the shock I felt when I saw the positive result appear for the first time. My head was spinning and I remember frantically ringing Rikki and making him come home because I physically couldn't wait another minute to tell him. He came straight home and we just stared at the test in shock, then we talked all evening about becoming a mum and dad, when the baby would be due, what we needed to do next. Looking back, it was an incredibly exciting but nerve-racking time. We've been taught to keep those first few weeks of pregnancy a secret for fear that something might go wrong or that the pregnancy might not be viable, and sadly the statistics say that one in four pregnancies end in loss. The difficult part is that the first trimester is the time when you are probably feeling your worst. It's when most of the dreaded symptoms – such as morning sickness, fatigue and the roller-coaster of emotions that hormones bring – kick in, and feeling like you can't tell anyone why you feel rough is difficult. .

In those first few weeks when I was pregnant with Archie, we chose to tell close family because the timing meant we could surprise them on Christmas Eve and Christmas Day, which was really special, but we didn't announce it to anyone else until after the twelve-week scan. I used to think that keeping your pregnancy a secret until you were past those first uncertain three months was the most sensible thing to do, but after personally seeing pregnancy from both the side of getting the gift of a healthy baby at the end, and also from the side of suffering a miscarriage, I can see the importance of discussing the losses we experience as well as the happy endings. But of course, it's an individual choice. You've got to choose what's best for you.

It can often look like everyone we know has only had successful pregnancies because those are the only ones you hear about. But behind the scenes, there may have been a much more challenging journey than appears at first glance. I honestly thank those women who have been brave enough to open up and talk about their miscarriages and baby loss. Some are friends and others are brave ladies I've followed on social media, but all helped me to realise that it is very common and helped me feel less alone when it happened to me. Maybe if we all felt able to be more open and share our early pregnancy symptoms and talk about our feelings and mental health, it would allow us to feel supported and less alone. But announcing a pregnancy in those early weeks will suit some and not others, so go with your gut and do what feels right for you.

As well as telling my close family, I also reached out to a friend that was a few weeks further along in her pregnancy and who had already announced it. It was one of the best things I did. I opened up about how I was feeling and having the reassurance that she had gone through the same emotions of feeling scared and worried she wouldn't be able to do it was such a relief. So, reach out. Whether it's to your partner, a family member, a friend or even a health professional, don't go through the first trimester alone, and get the support you need. You can do this! And by the time the second trimester rolls around you'll begin to feel so much better. Most women get a lot more energy back during this time and for me it was the most enjoyable part of pregnancy. Here are some of my favourite hacks I discovered whilst I was pregnant. I hope you find them useful!

The Button Hack

Your bump's beginning to grow and your clothes are feeling a bit tight and uncomfortable, but you're still not at the stage where you're buying maternity clothes just yet. Get a few months' wear out of your trousers and jeans with one simple thing: a hair band!

Grab a thin hair band and hook it through the buttonhole in your jeans or trousers, then connect it to the button without doing it up. This gives you extra room for your bump to grow and finally you can sit down comfortably again!

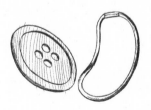

Ask for Help

Some of us find it hard to ask for help, but asking for some help while you're growing an actual human is not a weakness. In fact, at any point if someone asks: 'Is there something I can do to help you?' bite their hand off! Don't be proud and give them a job to do. Whether someone offers to make you a few dinners you can put in the freezer so that when baby arrives you don't have to worry about cooking, or they want to come over and do the vacuuming, they will probably feel great that they were able to do something for you as well.

Maternity Clothes

Being a mum doesn't have to mean that you lose your sense of personal style. Look at buying things that you'll still get some use out of after your pregnancy, such as buying sports bras instead of maternity bras or floaty dresses that fit with or without a bump. And get clever with accessories, such as bra extenders, in order to get the most out of the clothes you already own.

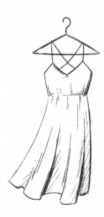

Get a Grabber

If you're getting to the stage in your pregnancy where you're finding it hard to bend down to pick things up off the floor or tidy up – especially if you already have kids and you're struggling to pick up their toys at the end of the day – get yourself a metal extended grabber, also known as a litter picker, to help you grab things you need, without having to bend down.

Pregnancy Apps

There are some fantastic apps that help you track your pregnancy. I personally loved that each week I could see how much the baby had grown and get a comparative size.

Some apps also show you a realistic 3D image of what the baby looks like as they grow each week and provide articles on the different stages of pregnancy and what you might be experiencing. I also found some great apps that help count your baby's (or babies'!) kicks during pregnancy, which is so important to keep an eye on, and also time contractions when the special day arrives!

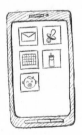

Eat Something Before You Get Out of Bed

Suffering with morning sickness can be one of the toughest parts of pregnancy, especially in the first trimester. Try keeping something light and plain, like crackers or ginger biscuits, by your bed so you can have one first thing in the morning before you get out of bed. This will help settle your stomach.

Newborn
Hacks

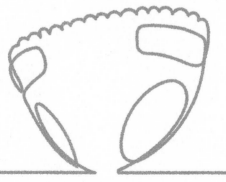

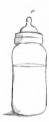

Congratulations! If you've reached this part of the book, then you may very well have a newborn baby in front of you right now. It's an incredibly special and precious time that I'm sure everyone you know is telling you will go by so fast. It's unfortunately the truest cliché I know. Whilst you know deep down how much you will look back and cherish this time, it can be hard to see the beauty of it through the fog of sleep deprivation and the overwhelming adjustment of life with a baby. As I said in my introduction, I was very naïve when I became a mum at twenty-four and had very little experience with babies. I had only held a couple of newborns in my life and had never changed a nappy or even changed a baby's outfit! It's true what they say, though: it does just come to you naturally and after the first few days, hours even, you learn and become more confident.

During those early days when you and your baby are getting to know each other, remember to go easy on yourself. Hormones begin flying around in the days after giving birth and the smallest thing can make you feel like you're getting it wrong or failing. It's all so normal and you and your baby are learning together. These are some of my most used tips and hacks to make life with a newborn run a little bit more smoothly.

The Vest Hack

I couldn't have got through the first night of being a new mum without this hack, and I'm so shocked at how many people have told me they didn't know this simple trick. So here it is: you can pull baby vests down over their shoulders instead of over their heads due to the stretchy envelope neckline you see on almost all baby vests.

This was an especially useful hack for us as my first son was very 'mucusy' when he was born and was sick about five times that first night in the hospital. (So don't let anyone tell you that you're taking in too many outfits – we got through them all and needed more!)

Aside from sick, this hack also comes in handy for poo explosions as it helps you keep the mess away from your baby's face, allowing you to change them with the least amount of upset for both of you and to keep things as clean as possible. The hack is also useful when your child gets to the wriggly, crawling-away-as-you're-trying-to-change-them stage as you can quickly pull the vest off them as they zoom in the other direction away from you!

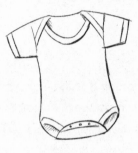

Watch Out for the Wee!

If you have a baby boy, you will probably, at some point, get weed on! Yes, I'm afraid it's inevitable. Something that I found really reduced the number of times this happened was to open up a clean nappy and place it under the dirty one as you lay them on their changing mat to change them. You can then quickly remove the dirty nappy and instantly have the fresh nappy ready to do up as soon as they are clean.

It can also help to gently rub a baby wipe across their tummy just before you change them as this sensation helps to encourage them to wee, so it goes in the used nappy before you take it off and doesn't end up on your only clean top!

The Breast-Feeding Basket

If you're planning on breast feeding, I always found it helpful to keep a stash of things in a basket close to my bed to help me get through the night feeds. My midwife even recommended eating a snack and having a drink during the night to help keep up my milk supply. Some of the things I would recommend having with you each night before you go to bed are a bottle of water and a quick snack, like a cereal bar, to give you a bit of energy and help to wake you up. You could also keep spare breast pads, nipple cream, tissues and wipes, and even the remote control if it's going to be a long night!

I bottle-fed my first son, but having some of the things mentioned above still really helped me get through those night feeds, especially in the beginning. It probably goes without saying that keeping another box or caddy full of nappies, wipes, muslins and a few spare baby grows and vests by your bed will alleviate the need to be up and down all night. And there's no doubt that the less you have to get up, the better and calmer it is for both you and your baby.

We also worked out quite quickly that a foam changing mat on our bed was a lot quicker than taking our new baby into their bedroom, putting them onto a changing mat and waking them up even more with the lights and sounds that involved.

The Disappearing Stain

Those first few months of poo explosions take a fair bit of getting used to! It's amazing how such a small person has the ability to destroy all of those beautiful white vests, baby grows and outfits that you lovingly washed and folded away, waiting until the day you could dress your baby in them! Then, no sooner do they have it on than it goes from white to a rather less attractive mustard shade! And sometimes, even after a few washes, that beautiful baby grow seems like a lost cause. Or is it?

The day I discovered that the sun is nature's way of bleaching stains, I felt like a genius. Place the washed item of clothing in the sun and watch the poo stains disappear. OK, maybe give it a few hours. But it'll happen! This works best on white clothing and it also works well on soft baby pinks and blues and

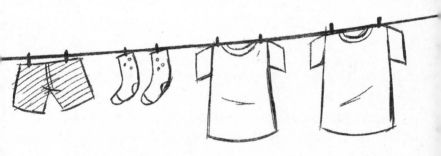

any pastel colours, as the sun bleaches out the stain. However, avoid anything too brightly coloured as you don't want the sun to bleach the vibrant colours too.

Neat Nails

As a new parent, cutting your baby's nails can seem like a daunting task. Those tiny nails on those tiny hands, that love nothing more than to flail about, are an impossible moving target. You might as well attempt to put mittens on an octopus! But cutting their nails is really important as, although they might be small, they can be sharp! And there's nothing worse than seeing your beautiful baby's face with scratches all over it.

After trying lots of different techniques, I've found that the best way to do it is to cut your baby's nails when they're asleep. Once your baby's nodded off, wait about twenty minutes as they'll be in a deeper sleep and it will be so much easier to cut their nails safely when they're not wriggling around. You can use a small lamp or even a torch pointed at their hands to make sure you can see what you're doing but not disturbing them. Lots of kits are available with all the tools you'll need, including baby scissors and even tiny baby nail files to make sure the edges are smooth.

Spare Top

Something I often forgot in the early days is that because new-born babies can be messy, that often means you'll be messy too! The amount of times we went out for the day and ended up with baby sick or poop on me is more than I care to remember. So, I always found it helpful to pack a spare top in the baby bag. This was also extremely helpful if ever there was a leaky boob situation as well!

It may seem like a no-brainer, but in those early days when baby brain has taken over and you have a million and one things to remember (I mean, let's face it, it feels like you need to pack everything but the kitchen sink just for a trip to the local coffee shop), it's all too easy to forget about what *you* need for the day too. Up next is a handy list of things, alongside a spare top, to pack when you go out for the day. For baby *and* for you.

WHAT TO PACK IN YOUR BABY BAG (NEWBORN TO SIX MONTHS)

I remember feeling really overwhelmed when I first thought about what I needed to pack in my baby bag. The paraphernalia that comes along with a new baby – just to be able to leave the house! – is impressive, and forgetting something important can be disastrous and send you running for the nearest supermarket. As a general guide, these were the things I would always have to hand in my baby bag, especially when mine were between the ages of zero and six months.

NAPPIES

A good rule of thumb is to take one for every hour you'll be out. It's better to be safe than sorry with nappies – no one wants to run out of those!

BABY WIPES

A full pack of wipes will be just what you need for a long day out. Make sure you're stocked up, as you'll probably end up finding packs in every corner of the house and car as time goes on because they come in so handy for lots of little things, both at home and out and about. As helpful as they are though, there's one thing they don't help and that's the environment. As we all become more mindful of the impact we are having on the planet, alternative options such as biodegradable and compostable wipes are great options that mean you can keep everyone and everything clean without the guilt!

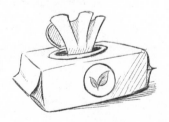

TRAVEL CHANGING MAT

Many changing bags come with a travel changing mat already inside, but if yours doesn't, I really recommend getting a travel changing mat, that way you only have to take your baby and the travel changing mat to the toilet with you. That way you can keep one or two nappies, baby wipes and some nappy cream inside and simply take your baby and changing bag to the toilet for a quick change. This is especially handy if you're somewhere that has tiny changing facilities.

NAPPY BAGS

There's nothing worse than when your baby has a poo explosion over one of their best outfits and you've forgotten to pack the nappy bags since they're the perfect portable dirty-laundry bag too. I would definitely recommend packing a roll in your bag so you always have them to hand. You can get many varieties including scented, antibacterial and biodegradable ones.

CHANGE OF CLOTHES FOR YOUR BABY

Depending on how long you'll be out, it's probably best to take a few outfit changes for your baby. They always seem to have an accident the minute you put them in that lovely outfit your friend bought them and has been dying to see them in! Some weather-appropriate clothes, a couple of vests and a sleep suit are good options since, if you're out when they would usually sleep or would be putting them to bed, they can be changed into night-time clothes to help them settle.

CHANGE OF CLOTHES FOR YOU

As discussed previously, don't forget a change of clothes or at least a clean top for you!

FEEDING SUPPLIES

These will vary depending on how you're feeding your baby. If you're formula feeding, then it's recommended that your baby should drink a bottle within an hour of it being made up. So, if you know your baby will be due a feed later on in the day, there are some other options. Baby powder dispensers are really handy: you can fill the compartments with pre-measured amounts of powder so you know your baby is getting the right amount. Some bottles also come with a small pot that you fill up with the correct amount of powder and place securely inside the top of the empty bottle until you're ready to use it, which is clever and space-saving too! If you need to make fresh bottles up on the go, the easiest way is with a Thermos flask of boiling water, as you need to sterilise the powder, and another bottle of cooled boiled water. You can then make your bottles up by adding the powder to the boiling water to kill any germs and then topping it up to the right level using the cooled boiled water. It should mean you have a bottle at the right temperature to feed your baby (always check first) straight away and you don't need to wait for it to cool down before you can feed them. Another alternative is to buy the pre-made bottles of formula which make it so easy as they are ready to use – these definitely helped us out as new parents!

If you're breast feeding, then you shouldn't need to take too many supplies with you. However, if you have expressed breast milk into a bottle to bring with you, then it's best to put it in a cool bag with an ice pack to keep it fresh.

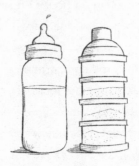

YOUR OWN BAG

I always found it easier to use the changing bag for my belongings as well as everything I would need for the baby. It's much easier than taking two bags everywhere with you. With that in mind I found a pouch, such as a make-up bag, the easiest thing to use. I would keep everything in there including my phone, keys, purse and lipstick so I knew where everything was and it was easily accessible. This is definitely easier than digging through the bag to find your phone, and the pouch took up less room than a normal bag too.

EXTRAS

It's easy to get carried away and feel like you have to pack everything except the kitchen sink, but keeping it simple and only taking what you think you'll need is key. With that in mind there may be extras you need as the weeks go on such as a dummy if your baby takes one and a dummy box (to keep the backup dummy in!) You might also want to bring your child's favourite toy or blanket. It's always easier if your baby's first travel toys attach to the pram or buggy to leave you room in the bag, but underneath your pram is another great place to store extra things such as a special comforter that they can't sleep without.

You might also want to keep a bottle of hand-sanitising gel and some antibacterial wipes in your changing bag, just in case. Often changing facilities aren't the nicest places and you'll be glad you put them in your bag, as well as some teething powder for when those pesky teeth start to cause them pain.

Outfit Organisation

A great hack I discovered after realising how many outfit changes a baby can go through in a day was to use a shoe organiser, the kind that you hang over the back of a door or inside a cupboard, to keep baby's outfits organised and together. Because they're so small, you can easily fit a baby vest or pair of leggings, for example, inside one of the pockets, and because they're clear you can see exactly what you've got. This way, instead of trying to put an outfit together when your baby's crying or mid-change, you can spend a bit of time putting the right combinations together when you have a spare ten minutes at home and then you can easily grab an outfit and go. This works especially well for soft fabrics such as wool and cotton because you can roll them up and they won't crease, leaving space in your baby's wardrobe or drawers for smarter clothes that they might only wear every now and then.

The Changing Mat Trick

As changing mats are generally made with a plastic or oil-cloth covering to make them waterproof, they can feel really cold when babies are placed on them, especially if they've come from a cosy cot straight onto the changing table. One trick you can use to make it more of a smooth transition is to place a bed pad or puppy training pad on the changing table before you lay them down. Not only does this mean they aren't suddenly shocked by the cold mat, but the absorbent material of the mat soaks up any accidents or sick which might – and let's face it, often does – happen whilst you're changing them.

Some nappy brands also have a coloured strip which changes colour once your baby has done a wee, so you can tell with a glance and don't have to disturb them too much if they're sleeping. This will save you having to move them to the changing mat unnecessarily!

White Noise

White noise works wonders for some babies. You can get soft toys that have white noise machines in them, and some of them also play heartbeat sounds to remind the baby of being in the womb, as well as nature sounds to help calm and soothe.

Not every baby is a fan though. My second son wasn't really keen, but I remember when we first tried it with my eldest, it sent him straight to sleep – it was like a miracle! He loves being sung to sleep even now so maybe some people just find it easier to drift off with a comforting sound.

Before investing in a white noise machine or toy, you can try it on an app on your phone, or even YouTube, which has eight-hour white noise videos. Household objects such as the hoover or hair dryer being used in another room also create white noise, so you could always try giving the bedrooms a clean or drying your hair whilst getting your baby to sleep – now that's what I call multitasking!

Changing Bag Bundle

If you want to utilise the space in your changing bag, make a baby clothing bundle. It's space saving and easy to take with you to the changing room. You simply lay your baby's outfit out – for example, a vest with a pair of leggings folded in half on top – then you lay a pair of your baby's socks on top with the openings sticking out. Roll everything up like a Swiss roll. You can then keep it neatly together, opening up each sock and wrapping them around each end of the bundle giving you a compact change of clothes that's easy to take out of your bag in a hurry.

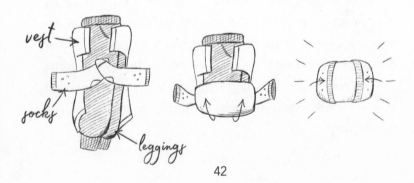

vest

socks

leggings

Changing Caddy

Make up a portable changing basket or caddy that you can keep downstairs with you and have close to hand. Having a nursery room with a changing table is lovely and looks beautiful but, practically, it's much easier to have enough supplies in the rooms you'll be spending most of your time in at home. You can fill it up every day with nappies, wipes, cream, spare outfits, toys and anything that you're using frequently at your baby's current stage. It saves you having to find things in different rooms and from running up and down the stairs all the time. I also found it was helpful to have a changing mat upstairs and one downstairs too – we used to keep it under the sofa as there was never a good place to store it – so it was easy to reach and we always knew where it was.

MAKING MEMORIES

When your baby is born, it all suddenly becomes clear that the cliché of 'it goes so fast' is sadly true. There are so many ways you can document the special moments and monthly milestones, which will become your most treasured keepsakes in years to come. Here are some of my favourite photo series ideas to remember those early months and years forever:

- A fun idea is to take a photo of them from birth in a nine- to twelve-month-old baby grow. At first it will completely swamp them of course, which will look really cute and funny, but as time goes on it will begin to fit them. It would be lovely to see how they've grown as they reach their first birthday.

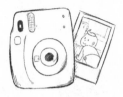

- Choose a special teddy and take a photo of your baby with it every month for the first year. Again, you will see how much they change and grow in comparison to the toy and that teddy will become a special keepsake too.

- Milestone cards: you can find many of these available pre-made now and they often have lots of other milestones that document special days such as 'First time I slept through the night' (always a celebration) and 'First tooth!' You could even make some yourself. Taking a photo of your baby with these cards is a lovely way to document the days these special firsts happened. You could then print them out and add them to a baby book with the date written next to it which would make a lovely gift for grandparents and family too.

- Another nice idea is to take a photo of you with your bump in the last few weeks of pregnancy then, once your baby is nine months old, put them in the same outfit as you wore and take a photo (preferably in the same place) to show your journey and your baby at nine months in and nine months out.

Sensory Box

As the weeks go on, you'll notice that your baby is able to better focus on objects, faces and lights. You can create some safe sensory toys for babies of all ages to provide enjoyable and stimulating activities for them.

Fill a box with household objects that have different textures or make different sounds, such as a rattle they can begin to grasp, brightly coloured or black-and-white objects, or pictures with bold patterns that will catch their attention and make them want to explore. You can also try filling up a bottle with water and glitter which is a great way to calm a slightly older baby – they'll be mesmerised by the colour and movement.

Email Address

We all know that it has become more and more difficult to secure your own personal email address with your name, as there are now so many people using the internet. Why not set your baby's email up for them now. You could send them funny messages, memories, photos and fun things they say that make you laugh, so that when you're both older they have a full inbox of emails from you that will be sure to make them smile.

Birthday Letters

If you prefer something a little more traditional, why not write a letter to your child on each of their birthdays, starting with the day they're born, and document their achievements each year. You could give them the letters in a beautiful book the day they turn eighteen. It would be such a genuinely heartfelt keepsake and something they would treasure forever.

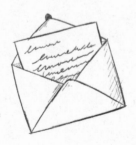

Swaddle Bathing

If your baby doesn't enjoy having a bath, try swaddle bathing. Swaddle them in a soft muslin first, then gently place them into their bath. Once they get used to it you can slowly remove the swaddle to clean them. Some babies really enjoy this and it doesn't come as such a shock as being suddenly placed in the water. It's a more gradual way to get them used to a bath in those first few months.

When we had our first son, we had a portable baby bath which we would fill up and put on the floor. We soon realised it was a lot of hassle and so heavy to lift. We found a soft mesh bath support so much easier. That way you can lower your baby into the bath without any heavy lifting and you have your hands free to clean them. They especially come in handy when you have more than one child and want to bathe your baby and a toddler too!

Birthing Ball Rocker

You may think the birthing ball is destined to be deflated and put in the loft once your precious bundle has arrived, but don't say goodbye to it straight away. Some babies love the motion of being gently bounced to sleep – after all, they were used to it when they were inside you, so it's a familiar, comforting feeling to them. Give it a go and see if your baby is a fan.

Zips for the Win

I can't tell you how many times I would be trying to do up the little poppers after a night-time change and, through bleary eyes, manage to connect them wrong, only to have to start all over again. It can be torturous when it's 3 a.m. and all you want to do is sleep. That's when I discovered zip-up sleep suits and it was life changing! They're definitely not as common as the regular popper design but more and more brands are selling them as demand grows. Something as simple as a zip can really save your sanity in the middle of the night when you haven't had much sleep and you're not really in the mood for a brain training exercise. They usually come with a small piece of fabric that covers over the zipper to stop it going near your baby's face too, so it's good to see, as time goes on, designs are getting smarter and more efficient.

Wind Whisperer

Winding a baby can be a long and laborious task. It's easy to think that the second your baby has finished feeding they need to be patted on the back to get their wind up, but this can often lead to fussy babies and sick-stained clothes for you.

Instead of putting your baby over your shoulder or patting their back to wind them, try gently sitting them on your knee with their back and head supported, lean them forward slightly and slowly move their body around in a circular motion. This always worked well for both of our babies and the wind came straight up! It felt so much calmer and gentler for them too.

Medicine

It can be quite daunting giving your baby medicine when all they've been used to is a breast or bottle. Especially if they have a high temperature and you've tried everything to get it down. Some babies just do not like taking medicine through a syringe or spoon at a young age. A handy hack for giving your baby medicine is to use the syringe that comes with most children's medicines, but dispense it through the teat of a bottle.

Making sure you have the correct dose for your baby's age, hold the lid of a bottle and place the tip of the syringe into the teat. As your baby starts to suck you can gradually push the barrel of the syringe and your baby will get the correct dosage of medicine. They should hopefully be less likely to spit it out or gag on the medicine because you aren't trying to introduce something they're not used to. As they get older and begin to get used to different ways of feeding and a variety of textures you can begin to use the syringe or a measured spoon on its own.

Lost Socks

No matter how hard you try, you always end up with odd socks and this is especially true for baby socks as they're so tiny. I honestly believe the washing machine eats them! Try putting all of your baby's socks in a mesh bag before placing them in the washing machine. This will keep them all together and stop you from hunting everywhere for the ones that have disappeared.

Weaning Hacks

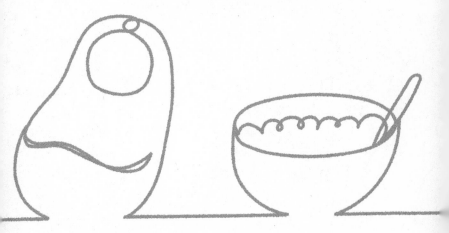

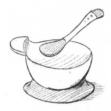

Weaning marks the start of a new chapter in your and your baby's life. It's a fun and exciting time and it's wonderful to see your little one reaching new milestones and having their first tastes of real food. But it can also be an anxious and confusing time for new parents as you begin to navigate the different ways to wean your baby. Weaning is recommended from six months and it's usually easiest to start with small amounts of vegetables, fruits and porridges. These can be puréed, mashed or, if you want to go down the baby-led weaning route, cooking the vegetables until they've softened is a good place to start.

I was so excited to start weaning my children. Trying them with a few new flavours and textures to start with and seeing the expressions on their faces as they discovered a new taste for the first time can be incredibly cute and hilarious in equal measures. Admittedly, it's a messy stage in your life, that's for sure. There will be lots of clean-ups, for you, your baby and the house – it's actually quite impressive how much of a mess one tiny person can make – but it's all part of the fun.

Here are some tips, tricks and handy products to get you started on your weaning journey. But remember, it should be an enjoyable experience for both of you. They say 'food before one is just for fun!' so don't stress if they don't like something. You can always try it again another time.

Crinkle Cut

Baby-led weaning is a great way to help your little one explore the proper texture and taste of food. But with tiny hands that are still learning to grasp, it's not unusual for babies new to the weaning game to struggle to hold certain foods, (most of which usually end up on the floor).

Try using a crinkle cutter to cut up your baby's cooked vegetables, and even some fruits. The ridges will give them a better grip on slippery foods. Try using this tip on carrots, sweet potatoes, melons and mangoes, to name a few.

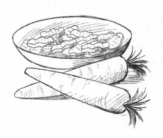

Keep It Handy

One of the not-so-fun things about weaning is the mess. It's something I used to struggle with but actually it's great for your baby's development and relationship with food to be able to touch, taste, smell and even play with it. A clever hack is to keep your baby's bibs close by by installing a sticky hook on the back of your baby's high chair. That way you can keep all the clean bibs together, you'll always know where they are, they are in easy reach and you can put one straight onto your baby as soon as they sit down to eat.

Grape Hack

One of the first tips I was given before I started weaning my first child is one that will always stick with me, and one that could actually save a life. Always remember to cut grapes and other small, round food, like blueberries or mini sausages, lengthways to reduce the risk of your child choking. It's a terrifying thought, but the shape of these foods makes them the perfect size to get stuck in a baby or child's throat.

Always remember to cut grapes down the longest part, and the same with sausages and anything else that you think may be a choking hazard. My children are past the baby and toddler stages now and I still do this and think I always will! A quick way to cut grapes in one go is to wash them and put them all on one plate, then turn another plate over and put it on top. Then with a sharp knife, slice between the two plates whilst holding down the top plate and voila! You'll have a full plate of cut grapes in seconds.

Homemade Porridge

There are so many baby products and foods you can buy for convenience now, but you can quickly and easily make your own baby porridge for a fraction of the cost of shop-bought baby porridge. It's a great first food because it can be mixed with their usual milk so it has a familiar taste with added texture.

Pick up a bag of regular rolled oats and blitz them in a food processor until the consistency is fine. Then add your baby's formula or breast milk and introduce different flavours such as puréed apple or mashed banana, depending on what your baby likes best.

HANDY WEANING PRODUCTS

Here are a few things I recommend buying when you start to wean your baby. As I mentioned earlier, it can be a messy job, and whilst it's great to embrace the mess as it's not going to be like this forever, there are definitely some gadgets out there that can make the process easier for everyone.

NON-SLIP SUCTION BOWLS AND PLATES

These are great because as the name suggests they stick to your baby's high chair or table with a suction pad, which stops plates from being thrown all over the floor or ending up on your baby's head. (Trust me, it's cute for a photo opportunity but after the hundredth time it gets a bit old!)

TEMPERATURE-SENSITIVE SPOONS

Such a clever idea. These spoons change colour when the food is too hot for your baby. Even though you would of course be blowing on your baby's food to make it cool enough for them to eat, as adults we're used to eating food much hotter than a baby can tolerate, so these are a really handy, visual way of telling when something is too hot. Even if you feel these aren't for you, a few silicone baby spoons are essential.

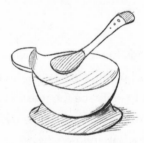

PLASTIC BIB WITH FOOD-CATCHER POCKET

I always found having a few plastic bibs so much easier as you're able to wipe them down after every meal and they're ready to use again, plus it saves on adding even more to your washing pile. The ones with the catch-all pocket on the front are great as well because, if I haven't mentioned it already, babies are messy. That way anything that would have landed on the high-chair tray or the floor, goes into the bib and makes clean-up so much quicker. You can also get long sleeved ones that are made of a waterproof wipeable fabric to completely protect clothes. Some even attach to the high chair, meaning there's no escape for any rogue food.

ICE CUBE TRAYS FOR FREEZING BABY PURÉE

Ice cube trays are a great way to store homemade baby food you want to freeze. That way you can pop out individual servings as needed. You can also buy purpose-made baby weaning trays which have larger sections and also come with a lid.

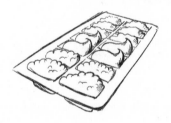

MESH FRUIT FEEDER

These are a fun way to introduce new soft foods such as strawberries to your baby. They usually look like large dummies and have either a mesh or plastic teat with holes in. You simply place the fruit inside the mesh part and your baby can chew on the dummy part to get the fruit out. If the fruit has been in the fridge it can also be quite smoothing for a teething baby with sore gums.

REUSABLE BABY POUCHES

If you want to make your own baby food but like the idea of the convenient pouches for purées, you can buy your own refillable ones. You fill them up from the bottom and seal them. Then they're ready to be used straight away or, depending on how long you want to keep them, you can store them in the fridge or the freezer, then when your baby has finished the food, you can wash them out and use them again.

OILCLOTH OR PLASTIC MAT

This is great to put under your baby's high chair at meal times. It's easy to wipe away any spillages and can be reused over and over again. It's especially handy if you have carpets you want to protect.

FROZEN LOLLY MOULDS

You can get specially designed ice-lolly moulds that are much smaller than normal ones, and designed for little hands to grip. They are great for turning your baby's favourite puréed fruits (and sneaky veg) into their very own ice lollies on a hot day.

Toddler
Hacks

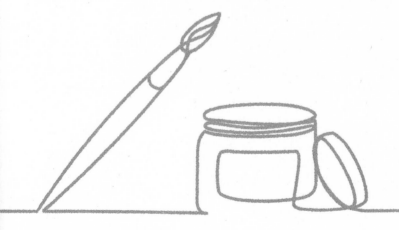

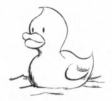

So you've reached the toddler stage. It doesn't seem like two minutes ago that your baby was a tiny newborn and suddenly they're crawling, standing and beginning to walk. At this age they start to become so headstrong and want some independence, but they still need so much help and support from you. I've often compared having a toddler to looking after your drunk friend on a night out when you're the designated driver. They're all over the place, bumping into things, falling over, they start to say some hilarious things, but can also be a bit temperamental and prone to a meltdown. It's a wonderful but exhausting time and just as previous challenges start to become a bit easier, new ones take their place. Here are some tried-and-tested hacks for getting through the toddler years in one piece!

Little Artists

Toddlers love to get creative and once they find their feet with paint, pens and drawing, you might find yourself with a rather large gallery of artwork from your budding artist. As time goes on, though, you might find that you have too much to display or put up on the fridge. A great a way to document all of your child's artwork without having to keep every single piece is to take a photo of it and keep it in an album on your phone. This way you can just keep the most special pieces, but you don't have to feel guilty about putting a few in the bin.

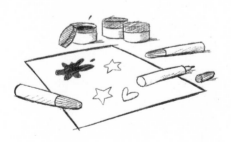

Kids' Cupboard

Little ones love to mimic what you're doing. If you need five minutes to start dinner or get something done in the kitchen, it's a great idea to have a cupboard or drawer full of safe children's play food or old pots, pans, bowls etc. that your child can play with to help keep them entertained while you get on with what you need to do. They will love feeling a part of what you're doing and it means you can keep an eye on them in the same room. If you have the space, having their own small toy kitchen nearby can give you a bit of time to cook or clean as well.

Bath Toys

Bath toys can get a bit grim over time. It's easy to clean the outside but often they have holes in them which you can't get to and mould can grow inside. To stop this from happening, when you buy a new bath toy, seal the hole up with a hot glue gun to create a waterproof seal that won't give mould a chance to grow.

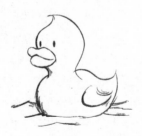

WHAT TO PACK IN YOUR TODDLER BAG (AGED TWO TO FOUR)

As my children got older, I found that I needed to take fewer things with us, which was amazing! I could actually start to carry my own bag again. I found the best bag to transition to was a child's rucksack. That way as your child starts to get older they can wear it on their back if they want to (although that usually lasts two minutes) and it means they can also use it for nursery, pre-school or a trip to their grandparents' house. Even though I class a toddler from the age of about one (or when they start to toddle around) I felt that the things I packed for my kids at the age of one to two were still almost identical to the baby bag – the only real change was the addition of food and feeding utensils. So, for the purposes of this list, I wanted to aim it more towards toddlers that are starting to potty train. Here's everything I packed in my toddler bag:

NAPPIES

If you're still at the start of your potty-training journey, it's a good idea to take some nappies with you as a backup. I would pack a nappy for every two to three hours you'll be out.

WIPES

These are always a must whatever age your child is! They come in so handy for so many things and, as well as toilet training, you also have messy toddler food and snacks to clean up. Again, as I mentioned previously, brands which make biodegradable wipes are becoming easier to find if you want to go down that route!

A CHANGE OF CLOTHES (OR TWO) FOR YOUR TODDLER

It's always best to take a few different outfits for your toddler with you until you are confident that they are dry throughout the day. And there can always be accidents or food spills, so it's good to have at least one clean outfit to hand. Try to pack things that are easy to take on and off, especially if you are encouraging them to use a potty or toilet whilst you're out.

TODDLER CUP

A good toddler cup can be hard to find, I lost count of how many we had that leaked, so a bag with an outside pocket that you can put the cup into could be really handy too. You want to look for one that is marketed as non-spill and the 360 cups where you have to suck to make the water come out are some of the best I've found, although they can take a bit of getting used to. Finding the right cup is a little bit of trial and error but once you do, you'll never look back.

FOOD AND SNACKS

Snacks are usually a toddler's favourite thing and their main priority in life. If you are going out around lunch time, and you want to be prepared with your own food from home, here are some of my favourite simple snacks to pack for toddlers:

- Raisins
- Chopped-up fruit
- Vegetable sticks
- Dried cereal
- Cereal bars
- Rice cakes

- Vegetable crisps
- Smoothie pouches
- Pita bread and dip
- Bread sticks

PORTABLE POTTY

You may not feel like venturing very far until you and your little one have nailed the potty training, so this definitely isn't essential, but it might be a good idea to take a portable potty with you and keep it in the back of the car for any longer trips.

EXTRAS

It's always worth making sure you're prepared with a few extras such as spare nappy bags for wet clothes and tissues for runny noses; and don't forget the antibacterial hand gel.

The Sticker Trick

As your toddler starts to get a little older and you want to give them more responsibility, like putting their shoes on, a clever hack to teach them which shoe goes on which foot is to cut a larger sticker in half and stick each half onto the inside of your child's shoes. This way, when they put them together, they can match up the picture and learn which is the right way to put their shoes on.

Super Surprise

Has your child ever had a lollipop and got bored with it within the first few minutes? Re-use old surprise egg cases (such as Kinder Eggs) as lollipop holders. Make a hole in the bottom of the egg big enough to slide the lollipop stick through and close the lid. That way, when you're out and about, if your child doesn't want to eat their lollipop all in one go or they want to play and run around and come back to it you're not left holding a sticky lolly.

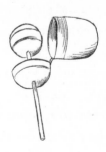

Clever Furniture

If you want to keep your home looking somewhat to your taste and have the ability to turn it back into an adult space when the kids go to bed, there are lots of great storage options and pieces of furniture you can buy that don't make your home look like a toy shop. Of course having toys around the house is part of family life, but it's nice to have the ability to hide it all away when they're not using them.

Baskets and trunks are great for storing toys. Trunks can also double up as side tables and coffee tables in the evenings and toys in baskets can be easily hidden away by adding a blanket or throw over the top. We love things like our wicker drawer unit that houses a lot of toys: it has ten drawers so it's easy to put things away in the right place. Even our built-in cabinets now mainly contain toys and puzzles instead of CDs and DVDs. Did I mention it's nice to be able to hide it all away and relax at the end of the day without stepping on Lego?

The Fifteen-Minute Rule

With toddlers, the smallest thing can set them off. Some of our excuses for not wanting to get ready have been: 'The jumper is too scratchy'; 'I need to wear my socks inside out'; 'The label's annoying me'. As a rule, I always try to give myself fifteen minutes more than I think I need before leaving the house. I mean, let's face it, we will probably still be late for wherever we need to be but by having a fifteen-minute buffer we end up *almost* on time!

Busy Box

A busy box is a great way to keep children entertained when you need a few minutes to get stuff done, or you want to sit down and engage in a fun activity together. It's great to fill these boxes with anything and everything you think could be made into something new, so whenever you're about to throw away a toilet roll tube or a milk carton, add it to the busy box instead. You could even add in some sticker sheets, paper and arts and crafts accessories such as pompoms and pipe cleaners. The best thing is that the creations will be different every time and the things you make will fuel your toddler's imagination. You can add to the box over time and because you're making use of junk and old packaging, it's a great way to reuse and recycle things too!

Busy Board

I love this fun idea to keep toddlers entertained. Have you noticed that your car keys, bag zip, door handles and door stops seem to be irresistible to your toddler? They love to get into things and see how they move and work, but often it's something you don't feel they should be playing with. If you or someone you know is a bit handy with the tools, you can create your toddler's very own busy board for little to no money.

Take a wooden board and attach items such as door knockers, zippers, wheels on castors, door chains, clips and anything that opens and closes or has an interesting texture or mechanism. You may even have many of these items around the house or in the garage or shed that you're no longer using. It's great to help toddlers develop their fine motor skills and will keep them busy for ages! I have seen some that are pre-made if you would rather buy one but it's fun to get creative and see what you can come up with.

Go Bag

A go bag is a similar idea to the busy box, but instead you can keep it in the back of the car and have it on hand for days out or restaurant trips. It could be a rucksack or handbag but instead of filling it with arts and crafts or junk modelling supplies you can put in toy cars or age-appropriate small toys. You can add in some stickers and some colouring books and crayons in case you go somewhere that doesn't supply them.

Why not also try making your child's own drawing pack with an empty DVD case. Children love little surprises and anything they can open to discover what's inside. Add some paper, crayons, pencils and stickers into an empty case, anything that's flat enough to fit inside. They could even create their own covers to put inside the front of the case. It's small and compact and easy to fit into a bag and you never know when it might come in handy.

Simple Sticker Sheets

This is a simple hack but one that comes in handy for little unco-ordinated hands. Whenever your child gets a new sticker book or sheet, peel off the surrounding borders leaving the stickers intact – it will make it so much easier for them to peel the stickers off.

Book Display

Using picture ledges or shelves, you can create beautiful, eye-catching children's book displays in their bedroom. Instead of having all of their books on a traditional bookshelf where you can only see the spines of the books, pick out their favourite books and create a library feel by creating a feature wall with as many picture ledges as you want. This is really engaging and makes it easy to see what books you have and means it's always fun to pick a book at bedtime. So many books have beautiful covers with brightly coloured illustrations, it's like creating your own art display! We've always done this and I love changing the books out for different ones to keep them interested. You could even style it to match the colours of your child's bedroom.

Cupcake Cases

Cupcakes cases have more uses than just baking. Take a paper cupcake case, make a small hole in the middle and slide it over an ice-lolly stick to create an ice-lolly guard! It helps to contain the mess and stops sticky lollies from melting all down your toddler's hands and arms.

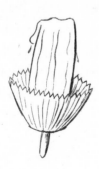

Play Wallets

As we know, children love nothing more than looking through a bag or a wallet, but they can often be filled with things you don't want getting into little hands, such as coins or medicine. Keep them entertained for ages with a wallet or bag of their own. You could fill an old purse or wallet with unused loyalty or membership cards, some paper or play money, a brush or empty, cleaned make-up cases or pots. They will have so much fun going through it, pretending to pay for things and acting grown-up like Mummy or Daddy. For slightly older children who are just learning to count, it could also be a great introduction to counting and maths and lead on to engaging role-playing games like shops and restaurants.

Non-Slip Baby Grows

As toddlers start learning how to walk and subsequently run around, albeit a little wobbly at first, baby grows and onesies can become a hazard as they can be quite slippery, especially on hard floors and surfaces. Many baby grows come with grippy soles as you begin to buy the larger sizes, but if they don't, add hot glue gun dots to the bottom to help give your little one some extra grip.

If your child is starting to grow out of their baby grows and you want to get a bit more wear out of them, you can cut the feet off the bottom to give them room to grow. That way you won't be buying so many, so it's better for the environment and your bank account, and it's another way to help them with their new walking adventure. Whilst we're talking about getting more wear out of things, you can also get vest extenders which fit onto the poppers that do up underneath, making the vests longer, and the great thing about them is they're reusable.

Backwards Baby Grow

Some toddlers get into a habit of taking off their baby grow or sleep suit and in turn taking off their nappy, which can obviously get extremely messy and not what you want before they are potty trained. If you can't seem to curb the problem, try putting their baby grow on backwards so it's harder for them to open.

Handy Handles

This is one of my favourite hacks and one that's saved a lot of juice-related spillages. Simply take a carton of juice, pull out the triangular 'wings' on either side and you have perfect, ready-made juice carton handles. No more grabbing hold of the carton and squeezing it everywhere. Trust me, once you try it, you'll never go back and you'll wonder how you lived without this trick before.

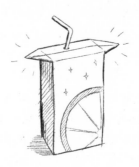

MESSY PLAY IDEAS FOR TODDLERS

Most toddlers love getting messy! They love anything with interesting textures and it can really help to develop their fine motor skills. Here are some of my favourite messy play ideas. NOTE: none of these are edible and children should always be supervised when making and playing with them.

Moon Sand

Moon sand is a fun sensory sand that's easy to make with just a few ingredients that you might already have at home. It holds its shape when rolled into a ball, pushed out of a mould or cut, but it also crumbles back into sand, so it's fun to create shapes and build things with.

You Will Need:

4 measuring cups of all-purpose flour
½ cup of baby oil or vegetable oil
A few drops of food colouring, optional

Method:

In a large mixing bowl, add all the ingredients and mix together until well combined and it looks like chunky sand but holds its shape when you squeeze it together. If it doesn't, add a few more drops of oil until it's the right consistency.

Cloud Dough

Cloud dough is another super easy activity you can create yourself at home and really wow your kids with. It's a silky, soft dough that you can roll, mould into shapes and cut shapes out of.

You Will Need:

2 measuring cups of cornflour
1 measuring cup of hair conditioner (any conditioner will work –
it gives this dough a beautiful scent)
A few drops of food colouring, optional

Method:

In a large mixing bowl, add all the ingredients and mix together until well combined and you have a solid dough. If you find that your cloud dough is still a little bit sticky, add small amounts of cornflour until you create a non-sticky consistency.

Bubbles

Who doesn't love a bubble? Best used outside, you can have hours of fun with your child, blowing bubbles and letting them jump and catch them. You can buy large bottles of pre-made bubble mixture and have fun using different objects to see what size bubbles you can make, but if you run out, it's easy to make your own at home.

You Will Need:
1½ cups of water
½ cup of washing-up liquid
2 teaspoons of sugar

Method:
In a medium bowl, add all the ingredients together and stir until combined. You can double or triple this to create thousands of beautiful bubbles.

Have fun finding objects around the house that you could use to blow the bubbles. You can create a homemade bubble wand with a wire coat hanger, pipe cleaners or plastic bottle with the bottom cut off. Or impress your toddler by making the bubble come straight from your hands! Simply dip your hand into the mixture, make a fist and slowly open your hand to make an 'O' shape and blow. (Elliot, my three-year-old, thinks this is amazing and he often asks me to do this with his bubble bath at bath time!)

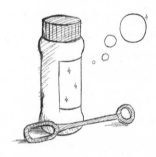

Squeezy Paint Dispensers

Keep hold of your old squeezy condiment bottles or hand and body wash dispensers that have a pump to create easy, squeezy paint dispensers. Once empty, wash them out and fill them with different coloured paints to make messy play a little bit cleaner.

If using dispensers with a pump, you can control the amount that comes out by wrapping the pump of the bottle with a hair band or elastic band so that it dispenses less paint at a time.

Pasta Play

A great way to explore different textures is with uncooked pasta shapes. You can put them on a large tray or even add some to an empty bath. In fact, the bath is a brilliant place for messy play as your child is contained and you can easily clean it out once you're done.

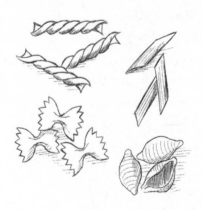

Rice Rummage

Fill an old container or plastic storage box with uncooked rice and hide different shaped objects inside for your toddler to find. They'll have great fun digging through and searching for their surprises. For older toddlers you could hide different shapes in the rice, which they have to find and sort into different shape categories.

If you want a similar idea with less mess you could create your own lucky dip box in a similar way but using shredded newspaper and toys or objects hidden inside. These can be toys from around the house and, for an added level of fun, you could wrap each one up to make the game last longer and feel even more exciting.

Spaghetti Worms

While dried pasta is a great option, you can also create hours of fun with your little ones by cooking up some spaghetti and playing spaghetti worms. Once cooked, leave to cool and then place inside a large bowl or storage box. Your toddler will love picking up the worms and exploring the look and texture. You could even add some food colouring to make them look more interesting.

Organising Hacks

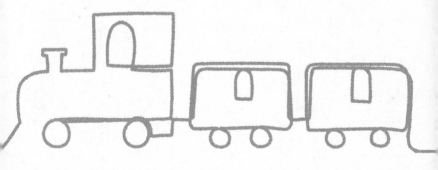

Organising
Hooks

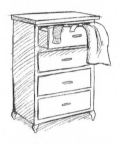

Now, don't get me wrong, my house is often in a mess. I've learnt over the years that with kids a mess is hard to avoid and to a certain extent you have to accept and enjoy the clutter and chaos. I really love seeing the boys enjoying their toys and I love that our house usually looks and feels very lived-in and family friendly. But, on the other hand, I really do love an organisation session. There is something about seeing a messy cupboard, drawer or room become tidy, clean and organised to perfection that is so satisfying, and if everything has its place then it's easier to keep on top of the day-to-day mess. I honestly feel like when the house is clean and tidy, my brain is that bit clearer as well. And if you can just push past the 'I wish I never started this' stage, then you feel such a sense of pride. No one wants to have their cupboards piled high with clutter or to have to struggle to find what you need, so here are some of my top tips for keeping your home organised.

Stair Basket

We always find we end up piling things on the stairs that need to go up and then everyone just walks past it. So a nice stair basket is really handy. You can fill it up throughout the day and then just take everything up with you in the evening and put everything back where it belongs. They usually come with a cut-out section that sits around the shape of a step and you can get beautiful wicker and rattan ones to suit your home decor.

Making the Bed

Making the bed every morning is a great way to tick something off your to-do list and motivate you for the day ahead. I must admit though, putting on clean sheets is not one of my favourite jobs. Years ago, I learnt this clever hack to make it so much easier and I've put clean bedding on this way ever since.

The simplest way to put on a clean duvet cover is to turn it inside out, put your arms inside the cover and into the top two corners then, with your hands still inside the duvet cover, grab the top two corners of the duvet and shake the duvet cover down over it, which will now be right side out. Give it a shake, do up the buttons and it's done. Honestly, I haven't made the bed differently in about fifteen years!

Pillow Pockets

Keep your bedding organised and easy to find by storing each set in a matching pillowcase. Fold up the duvet cover, sheet and the rest of the pillowcases and put them inside, making it easy to store neatly in a cupboard and easy to grab when you want to make the bed.

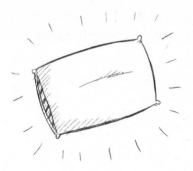

Tumble Dryer Sheets

Even if you don't own the machine, tumble dryer sheet have lots of uses around your home aside from the obvious (adding them into your tumble dryer). They have a lovely, fresh scent that lasts for ages, so once you've finished organising a linen cupboard or clothing drawer, put them inside to make your clothing smell nice. You can also put them inside cushion cases, so you get a nice scent when you sit down on the sofa, in car doors, or pop a few in the shoe cupboard to keep bad odours at bay.

Start Small

If you want to get organised but you don't know where to start, start small. It could be one drawer or cupboard per day. Give yourself ten minutes on a timer and see how far you get. It's amazing how quickly you can sort out a kitchen drawer that you've been struggling to close for months or a shelf in the airing cupboard when you've got a focused amount of time to get it done. It will also give you such a sense of achievement once you've done it – you'll be more likely to carry on and do another drawer and another!

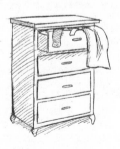

Don't Forget the Door!

Don't forget to utilise the space you have on the backs of doors and cupboards. It's such a handy and sometimes unused space as once it's closed it's hidden away. You can keep shoe organisers on them – to make sure your shoes are stored together and not just thrown into the bottom of a cupboard or wardrobe – or you can use them to store a multitude of other things. Spice racks that screw on to back of kitchen or larder cupboard doors are a great use of wasted space. Door hooks are perfect for storing dressing gowns behind your bedroom door and many hook over the top of the door so you don't have to damage it. Accessory organisers, such as jewellery and belt hangers, can be added to the inside of wardrobes so you can easily display what you have and see everything at a glance when choosing what to wear for the day. Lots of things that would get thrown to the back of the drawer can easily be organised by using wasted space on the back of the door.

Lazy Susan

These spinning dividers are a great addition to a cupboard to utilise the space and help you to see what you have instead of leaving things to go out of date in the backs of cupboards. They're great for storing cans and bottles in a kitchen cupboard, but they also work great for beauty and hair products in a bathroom cabinet, or stationery supplies in a home office.

Vacuum Pack Bags

Vacuum pack bags are a handy way to store large, bulky clothes or textiles that are taking up too much space. Items like spare duvets and cushions can be added to the bags and sealed up. Then with a vacuum you can remove the air from the bag, making the items inside smaller and easier to store under the bed or in a loft. They're really handy for storing out-of-season clothing as well, and have the added benefit of keeping them protected from dust and mould.

Drawer Dividers

Drawer dividers are a simple way of stopping a drawer becoming a junk drawer by separating your drawer into smaller compartments to keep it organised. Dividers come in all different shapes and sizes and you can get expandable dividers and trays to suit any drawer. They can be used for anything from organising underwear and socks to categorising make-up by type, organising kids' toys and giving the junk drawer in the kitchen a new, organised lease of life with places for batteries, tea lights, pens and whatever else tends to end up in there! You could even recycle old shoe boxes, gift boxes and packaging that you've saved to create drawer dividers too.

Battery Hack

Do you have a box of batteries but have no idea if they're used or not? Maybe you've found a few at the back of the junk drawer? An easy way to tell if a battery is fresh is to drop the bottom of it onto a hard surface from a height of about six inches. If it hardly bounces and then falls over, it's fresh. If it bounces a couple of times before falling over, it's either dead or been used before, which means it probably doesn't have much charge left.

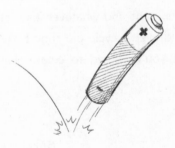

Folding Fun

Folding your clothes in the famous Marie Kondo way is more than just a fad. It's a fantastic way to optimise space and allows you to see exactly what you have. Instead of stacking piles of T-shirts on top of each other in neat, folded piles that you then mess up by trying to find a certain T-shirt at the bottom of the pile, you fold everything into neat parcels that stand on their own and fit nicely into the drawer, more like a filing system. It takes a bit longer to do when you're initially organising a drawer, but I find it ends up staying organised for longer and I get more wear out of my clothes because it's not as easy to forget about things at the bottom of the drawer. Check out Marie's book *The Life-Changing Magic of Tidying Up* to learn how to do this.

The Thirty-Second Hack

I believe that half the battle in keeping things organised is to do small jobs as you go throughout the day. If something is going to take you thirty seconds to do, do it straight away. It can be really easy to let things build up during the day to the point they become overwhelming and seem like a huge job in the evening. You can re-train your brain to do small, quick jobs as you go and you'll find that everything seems more manageable. So, next time you look at something that needs doing, ask yourself: Will it take thirty seconds? If yes, do it now – you'll be grateful you did, later.

Cleaning Hacks

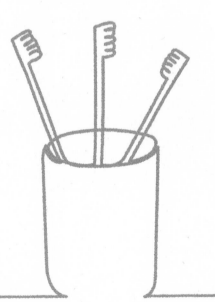

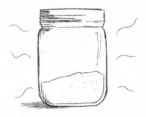

Cleaning. A seemingly never-ending job once you have kids. It can sometimes feel like you spend your whole life cleaning, just to turn round and see a scene of destruction behind you. Then the process starts again. Cleaning isn't my favourite thing to do but having a clean house is so rewarding. We aren't perfect but in our house we have found there are certain jobs we need to do every day in order to keep the house running smoothly, and if it's left for any longer then it gets a bit out of control and becomes a much bigger job. Something I feel really helps motivate me to clean is to use it as a time to also do something I enjoy. Whether it's listening to a favourite podcast, audiobook or album, there is plenty you can do to entertain yourself whilst doing those mundane tasks. Multitasking at its finest!

Upstairs, Downstairs

Most of us keep our cleaning products under the sink, but something I realised while raising my first child was that many of the products I kept there weren't even used downstairs – for example, toilet cleaner and carpet spray. These were things I only really needed upstairs, so I decided to have two dedicated cleaning caddies for each floor, and I store the upstairs products in a high cupboard upstairs. That way, I know everything is easy to reach depending on what I need for each room.

Also, while we're on this point, I've found that if I'm doing a whole house clean, it works better if I start upstairs and move downstairs, so that I'm not walking any dirt from downstairs back up. I also try and start at the top of the room so, for example, I'll dust anything up high, or on shelves, first and then dust and clean anything at mid-height such as on sideboards or bedside tables and finish by vacuuming the carpet or washing the floors, so any dust or dirt that has fallen down will be cleaned up last.

Dishwasher

To stop small items such as metal straws and small spoons from falling down into the bottom of the dishwasher, use a mesh bag to keep them all contained. The dishwasher is great for disinfecting things too so it's also a good method if you want to wash a load of small, plastic toys (ones that don't have batteries).

There are, however, certain things that shouldn't be put into a dishwasher. Most items will say on the base if they are dishwasher safe or not, but here is a list of a few more items you might not realise are *not* dishwasher safe:

- Sharp knives (washing them in the dishwasher can make them dull)
- Non-stick pots and pans
- Wooden spoons
- Crystal (such as crystal glasses etc.)
- Hand-painted items

- Chopping boards
- Insulated mugs and travel cups

When placing cutlery into the dishwasher basket, don't group the same utensils with each other, otherwise they can nestle together. Remember, 'spoons spoon' so when placed in the same slot they won't clean as well. Some dishwashers have individual slots for each item of cutlery, which means they all need to face upwards, and if you do choose to put sharp knives in the dishwasher, place them lying down in the top tray. If you still have your manual, it should tell you how to stack items in your model of dishwasher.

Microwave

To keep your microwave sparkly clean, add some water and lemon juice to a microwave-safe bowl. Set the timer for three minutes and put it on. As it's heating, the water will turn into steam and with the help of the citrus it will loosen any grease, grime and food residue so you'll easily be able to wipe it away.

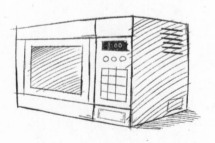

Fridge

Fill a glass jar with bicarbonate of soda and place it at the back of your fridge to absorb any bad smells and keep your fridge smelling fresh. It really works and you just have to change it every few months.

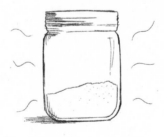

Venetian Blinds

I used to spend a long time trying to clean our Venetian blinds and shutters with special microfibre dusters designed to get into each slat, but the quickest and easiest way I've found to clean blinds or shutters is to simply close them! Then you have a flat surface to run your microfibre cloth over. You can usually tilt the slats both ways to clean both sides and it's really fast and easy.

Dryer Sheets (Again)

There seems to be no end to clever uses for dryer sheets. Because they help control static and lint, they're great for dusting. They pick up hair and dust but they also leave behind a residue that can make it easier to clean and stops dust building up again. As I've mentioned before, they also have the added benefit of smelling really nice!

Toothbrushes

Don't just throw away old toothbrushes, they're great to repurpose as cleaning brushes to clean small areas that are hard to reach, or narrow areas you want to clean, such as cleaning grout in the bathroom or dust from your computer keyboard. They also work great for cleaning things like shower door runners which can be hard to get into but can build up with a lot of soap scum. They really are very handy to have in your cleaning kit – just be sure to put them away in the cleaning cupboard so no one accidentally mistakes it for their current toothbrush!

Make It Sparkle

If your jewellery is looking a little bit dull, try adding it to a bowl with warm water and washing-up liquid and leaving to soak for twenty minutes. This mixture is great for gently cleaning jewellery made from silver, gold, platinum and precious gemstones. After it has been left to soak, go over it with a soft bristled nail brush or toothbrush to make it look as good as new.

Chewing Gum

This is such a pesky foodstuff and can be really annoying if your child's clothing or hair comes into contact with it. Here's how to manage both of those situations:

Clothing: A simple and easy way to remove chewing gum from clothing is to freeze it. You can either pat the area with ice cubes or leave the item in the freezer. Once the chewing gum has frozen and gone hard you can peel it off the garment. If any gum hasn't come off, use a dull knife to scrape off any remaining chewing gum and wash as normal.

Hair: To remove chewing gum from hair, don't rush to the scissors! Before taking any drastic measures, try removing it with oil (any oil such as olive oil, vegetable oil or coconut oil will work), as it breaks down the gum. First, section off any hair that isn't affected by the chewing gum and keep it out of the way. Then, over the bath or in a large bowl, apply a generous amount of oil and work it into the hair. The gum should begin to slide off the hair and you can brush out any small pieces with a comb. Once it's fully removed wash your child's hair a few times to remove the oil.

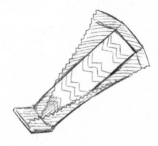

Laundry Hacks

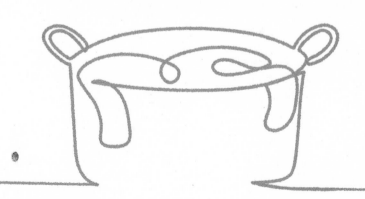

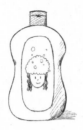

Another seemingly never-ending task is the laundry. No matter how many loads I do I rarely see the bottom of the laundry basket! It's something we try to keep on top of and do at least one load of washing each day to keep the pile as low as possible. My children, especially my youngest, Elliot, feel the need to get changed multiple times a day. I once counted seven outfit changes! Most of which I promptly put back in the wardrobe because they're not dirty! But during so many stages, from the newborn days of poo explosions and projectile vomiting to potty training, where accidents are inevitable, we end up getting pretty well acquainted with the washing machine! Let's talk stains (and not just on clothes!), symbols and smells.

HOW TO REMOVE STAINS

Stains are an inevitable part of any parent's life, so here are some tips for removing some of the most common ones I've come across.

CRAYON ON THE WALLS

Apply a small amount of toothpaste to the crayon mark and rub the stain with a cloth. Or for an even simpler fix, a magic eraser sponge will remove the crayon straight away. They're slightly abrasive so they work wonders to remove scuffs from walls and even those left in the bath from bath toys which seem impossible to remove.

OIL STAINS

For oil-stained clothes, rub some chalk into the stain and allow the chalk to absorb the oil. Wash as usual.

SWEAT STAINS

Sweat stains can be really hard to remove. Create a paste by adding a tablespoon of baking soda to a bowl and adding warm water until you get a paste-like consistency. Apply to the stain and let it sit for thirty minutes. Wash as normal. For older stains, try covering the stain with distilled white vinegar and leave to sit for thirty minutes before washing as normal.

MAKE-UP

Apply shaving foam onto the stain, add some cold water and work it in with a toothbrush. Wash in the machine as normal.

GRASS STAINS

Soak the stain with some distilled white vinegar. Then apply your laundry detergent straight on the stain and work it in. Wash in the machine on a cold wash.

FELT-TIP PEN

If your little angel has decided to create an original work of art on your carpet or sofa, use hairspray to lift the stain. Simply spray the area with hairspray and blot the mark with some paper towel. Keep applying until the entire stain has been removed.

Washing Machine Symbols and What They Mean

Before we get stuck in to the laundry tips that will change your life, it's really important to know what the symbols on your clothing mean, which I must admit, I wouldn't have known before becoming a mum! But there's nothing to be ashamed of, so if you need a little reminder, here's a list of all the most common ones and what they mean:

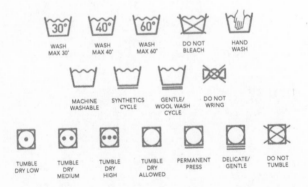

No More Mould

The washing machine is probably one of the most used items in your house. It's so important for keeping the whole family's clothing clean and smelling fresh, but we probably don't give enough time to making sure we're using it or taking care of it properly.

To help prevent mould and mildew from building up inside your machine, leave the washing machine door open for a while after you've finished a load, to give it a chance to dry. You can also do the same with the drawer. This will help with the build-up that you usually get inside the drawers and inside the washing machine seal.

Avoid Overloading

Overloading the washing machine can be very hard to resist when you only have a few more items to get clean, but it actually reduces the quality of the wash and doesn't clean your clothes as well. Always make sure you have left enough room in the washing machine for the water and detergent to circulate the clothes evenly. You can check this first by putting your arm into the machine and making sure there is space at the top.

No More Dye Dramas

Turn denim and brightly coloured clothes inside out. This will help keep the colours from fading and stop the dye transferring onto your other clothes. I also like to use a colour-catcher sheet too.

Order Matters

Add the laundry pod, gel or detergent and the fabric softener to the machine before putting the clothes in. This helps the cleaners do their job properly as they start to work as soon as the water fills the machine, and stops them sitting or getting caught up inside your clothes.

Clothing Revival

We've all lost clothes to shrinkage, but with this little tip you can bring most items back to life. All you need is a large bowl filled with lukewarm water, add in one tablespoon of regular hair conditioner, and mix it around so it disperses in the water. Then take the item and place it in the water and leave to soak for thirty minutes. After it has been soaked take the item out and wring out any excess water. Lay it on a dry towel and begin to reshape whilst still wet. Try to pull each area into shape as evenly as possible. Then let it hang to dry and voila! Your or your child's favourite item is ready to go back into the wardrobe to wear again.

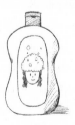

Deep Clean

Every six months, it's good to give your washing machine a deep clean. We often forget that items in our home that we rely on to clean need to be cleaned themselves in order for them to work their best.

To give your washing machine a deep clean, start by emptying out the filter. You can do this by laying down some old towels and either draining the water through the hose into a container, or if your washing machine doesn't have one, unscrew the filter and let that drain out into a shallow dish or tray. You might need to be ready with an empty one depending on how full it gets. If the filter itself is dirty, clean it well with hot soapy water before putting it back. Then you can move on to cleaning the drum.

Add 2 cups full of baking soda to the empty washing machine drum and run it on a hot wash for the longest time setting your machine has. Once finished, add 2 cups of distilled white vinegar into the drum and run the machine on another long, hot wash.

You could also add some drops of essential oil with the vinegar if you want to.

To clean the rubber seal of the washing machine, take a few tablespoons of baking soda and pour that inside the seal. Add in some white vinegar, enough to make the soda froth up but not spill out. Leave to work for ten minutes. Then give it a good clean-out with a damp cloth or an old toothbrush for any harder to reach areas.

You can also take the dispenser drawer out and soak it in some hot water and washing-up liquid in the sink to get rid of any product build-up or mould. If this doesn't remove everything, then you can create a paste with white vinegar and baking soda. Take half a cup of baking soda and gradually add the white vinegar until you have a paste, then work that into the tough areas with an old toothbrush. Finally, put everything back together and give the outside a clean with your usual surface spray or, again, for any difficult marks the same baking soda and vinegar paste. Wipe any access off with a damp cloth and you will have a sparkling clean washing machine that gets your clothes looking as good as new.

Dryer Sheet Alternative

If you're lucky enough to have a tumble dryer, I've learnt some brilliant hacks over the years that have been game-changing. If you want to try an alternative to dryer sheets and swap them for something reusable and easily recyclable, why not try balling up a couple of tinfoil balls and adding these to your dryer for the next load. The balls of foil channel electrons that positively and negatively charge each other, so it stops your clothing coming out of the dryer with static cling.

Tennis Tumble

You can use a tennis ball in your tumble dryer to help evenly dry larger items that sometimes don't come out fully dry such as duvet covers and sheets. You know when the bedding has been in the dryer for a while and it's mainly dry apart from a few annoying patches that are still damp or wet? A tennis ball will help move the items inside around and dry them more evenly. The only downside is it can be a bit noisy.

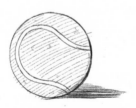

Quick Dry Trick

If you forgot to take something out of the washing machine to dry it the night before and suddenly panic that it needs to be worn the next morning, take a clean towel and add that into the tumble dryer with the wet clothes. This will help it dry much faster.

Easy Steam

Often I find that if I take things out of the dryer as soon as the load has finished and pull and flatten them back into shape, they usually come out crease free, but some items are just more prone to creasing. So why not try steaming them in the dryer. All you need to do is add a few cubes of ice to the dryer and when the heat of the dryer meets the ice it creates steam, helping to remove creases from your clothes. This works best in a smaller load, so if you're bored of ironing, give this a go on a few shirts and save yourself a job!

MY CLOTHING HEROES

I like to have a little box of helpful tools that keep our clothes looking as good as possible. It's surprising how much wear you can get out of something by fixing certain problems yourself instead of throwing it away (plus this is so much better for the environment).

DE-BOBBLER

I love our de-bobbler. It's a little battery-operated machine that you run over the surface of clothing that has gone bobbly, especially great for items like school jumpers. The small blade inside gently takes off the bobbles leaving it looking as good as new.

LINT ROLLER

We have one of these in the downstairs cupboard ready to use before we leave the house. Having pets can often leave you covered in hairs before you've properly started the day, so before we go out, we roll our clothes down and the hair is gone. We also keep one in the car and I have sometimes had a travel one for my bag, although they're hard to find. You can pick up the regular lint rollers with the sticky paper in most supermarkets and discount shops, but you can also get reusable lint rollers which have a sticky gel surface. You roll it over the clothes as usual to remove the hair and then wash away what it has collected under the tap. Leave to dry and it's sticky again.

STEAMER

I'll be honest, I'm not the biggest fan of ironing. (Does anyone truly love it?) I always seem to make things more creased than when I started, but since investing in a steamer I haven't looked back. I absolutely love how quick and easy they are to use. I just hang each item on the door and within a minute the wrinkles drop out before your eyes. I usually find it leaves clothing looking so much smarter and more presentable.

SEWING KIT

It's always good to have a little sewing kit to hand for emergencies, as you never know when a button will pop off or a hole will appear. I also keep some safety pins in ours in case I want to make a dress not quite as low cut, for example. Keep any spare buttons that come inside clothing in the box too so that if one does come off you know exactly where to find the spare ones.

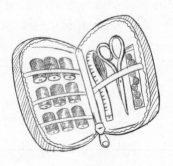

Clever Boot Warmers

A great way to reuse old jumpers you no longer want is to turn them into boot warmers for the whole family when it gets cold. Instead of giving away or throwing out damaged jumpers, save any with large, baggy sleeves. Just cut the sleeves off, then wear them over your socks inside a pair of long boots or wellies for extra toasty warm legs.

Smelling Fresh

To help keep your laundry basket smelling fresh and clean, take something like an organza bag or an old pair of tights, fill it up with baking powder and ten drops of your favourite essential oil and secure tightly. Then keep this at the bottom of the basket or bag. The baking soda will help to remove the bad odours whilst the essential oil will give off a nice smell.

Kitchen Hacks

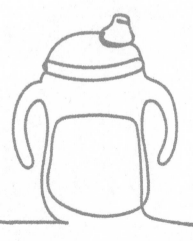

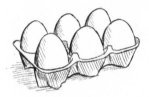

I'm always looking for ways to make my life simpler in the kitch-en. It can be really difficult to come up with new and interesting meal ideas that are healthy and that the whole family will eat. In fact, that's often an impossible task! With a busy family life, especially when everyone is at home, it can end up feeling like you spend your whole day making meals for everyone. Here are some of my favourite hacks to save yourself time and stress when it comes to all things food!

Meal Planning

Meal planning is a great way to get organised for the week. The day before we do the food shop, either online or in store, I make a list of the days of the week that we will be at home and browse through recipe books, cards and websites to find some inspiration. I'll also look in the cupboards and fridge to see what we have and how I can incorporate anything left over or that keeps for longer in the cupboards into next week's meals so things don't go to waste.

I'll also save the recipes we're using and write down the ingredients I need so I have it all in front of me when I'm doing the shopping. I do this mainly with dinners as that's usually the only meal the whole family is at home for, but you can get as organised as you like and create a meal plan for breakfast, lunch and dinner if you want to! I find that it helps to keep it interesting, as I spend a bit more time finding new recipes when I have time to sit down and concentrate, but it means that during evenings when we're in a rush getting in from school and nursery, or in and out to after-school clubs, I don't have to worry about what we're going to eat. I just have to put it all together.

Clever Cup

If you find yourself washing dozens of cups a day, add a magnet onto the back of a plastic cup which can be stuck to the fridge so your kids know where their dedicated cups are. They can then be refilled throughout the day, washed out and put back on the fridge when they're not being used.

Pancake Pourer

To make pancake mixture pouring much easier, simply mix up your pancake mix and add it to a clean, empty bottle (the squeezy kind that condiments come in would work best!) Then you can easily squeeze it into the pan and save lots of mess. This will also make it a lot easier to create some fun pancake art if you fancy! If you don't finish it all you can store it in the fridge for up to two days and use the rest the next day.

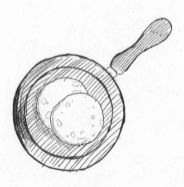

Fruit in a Flash

A super simple way to remove the core and stem of a strawberry is by pushing a straw up through the bottom of the strawberry. It's easy to do and means that you hardly waste any fruit. Likewise, sometimes peeling an orange can get a bit fiddly or just takes up more time that you would like. If you want the quickest way to prepare an orange just cut off the very top and bottom, and then cut down the middle of the orange about a quarter of the way until you're able to unroll the strip of orange segments.

Eggspert

Check to see if an egg is still edible by filling up a bowl or pan of cold water and popping the egg in. If the egg sinks to the bottom then it's good to eat; if it floats it's time to bin it. You can also easily separate the yolk from the white by taking an empty plastic bottle and squeezing it, then when you begin to release it again, hold the neck of the bottle over the yolk and the suction will pull it into the bottle, where you can then squeeze it gently back out into a different container or bowl.

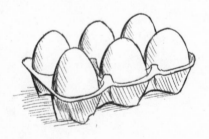

Potato Peeler

If, like me, you really despise peeling potatoes, try this hack: score a line around the middle of each potato, just enough to cut through the skin, then boil them with the skin on for fifteen to twenty minutes, depending on the size of the potatoes. Once boiled, remove the water and cover them again with cold water for five minutes. Once you're able to pick them up, rub your hand across the potato and the skin will begin to fall straight off. No more potato peeler needed!

Keep It Cool

If your child takes a packed lunch or a water bottle to school, try this simple hack to keep their drink colder for longer. Fill a drinks bottle half of the way full and put it in the freezer. The next morning, take it out of the freezer, top the rest of the bottle up with water and add it to your child's bag. It will stay nice and chilled, but they can also start drinking it straight away as it's not fully solid.

Morning
Hacks

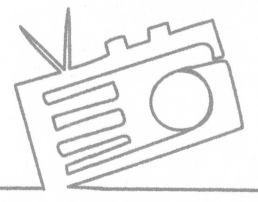

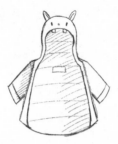

Often the most stressful part of the day is getting everyone up and out of the door in the morning, remembering the 101 little things you need to do or pack for the kids along the way. For me, getting organised begins the evening before, because as much as I think I'll be able to get it all done in the morning, it only takes a few things to go wrong – like a missing school jumper or a toddler tantrum – to throw everything off and make you late. I'm speaking from experience here as this has happened many times! Even if you're not a morning person there are routines you can put into place to make them much more enjoyable and less stressful. Here are some ways to make your mornings run a little smoother.

Get Ready Chart

If you have slightly older kids who are beginning to learn to do things for themselves, create a morning routine chart so children know what they need to get done each morning before school. This way they can learn what their responsibilities are and it also frees up more time for you. You can make them in lots of different ways, but here are a couple of ideas:

- Laminate an A4 piece of paper. Print off some images, or find them in magazines, that show your child's responsibilities – such as brushing teeth, eating breakfast and getting dressed – and then laminate them and cut them into circles. (The pictures are good for children that aren't reading yet.) Stick a piece of velcro to the activity and to the chart so that they can reuse it every day by sticking the activity onto the chart when they've completed the task.

- If your children can read, you could make each of them a pot filled with wooden pegs that say each of their morning jobs. Once they have done a job, they can clip the peg to the side of the pot and when they're at school you can put them back in the pot, ready for the next day.

After a while you'll find that they get into a routine and do these jobs each morning as second nature and won't need the prompt any more.

Keep It Together

I really do love a shoe organiser, especially to store everything we need before we head out of the door. Having one in the downstairs coat cupboard means you don't have to search around the house for things. Fill up each pocket with everything from gloves and hats in the winter to sunglasses and sun cream in the summer. A pack of baby wipes, car keys, wallet, hand gel, a hairbrush, your perfume and aftershave, and even the dog leads can fit in a shoe organiser. Everything is easy to see, tidy and accessible.

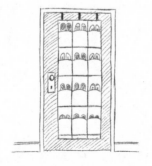

Save Time

Social media can be a huge time-sucker. I try not to look at my phone until I'm back from the school run so I don't get distracted by emails or social media. It's a good habit to keep you focused in the morning. It's easy to quickly go onto your apps and check what the rest of the world is up to even before you've properly started your day, and before you know it, twenty minutes are gone. Set yourself a time and don't go on it before then.

Mood Music

Something we try and do when we're not feeling the early starts or cold mornings is to put music on as soon as we get up. We like to listen to happy, upbeat music and it really does lift your mood and starts your day off on a good foot. Sometimes the simplest things are the most effective and we don't realise how much music can affect our mood. Put on your favourite radio station or playlist as soon as you get up, and you'll soon find yourself having a dance around the kitchen whilst you're making breakfast. I also find this works better to keep everyone focused on getting ready for the day because it's not as distracting as having the TV on but creates a good atmosphere. You can find lots of uplifting and motivating playlists on Spotify which have already been put together for you, but here is a list of some our favourite songs of all time and ones that always make me feel good.

OUR FAMILY'S TOP 10 TUNES

If you're stuck for inspiration on what to listen to in the morning, here is our family list. There's also space on the next page for you to add your favourite tunes.

1. 'Ain't No Mountain High Enough' – Marvin Gaye, Tammi Terrell
2. 'Always Be My Baby' – Mariah Carey
3. 'Rather Be' – Clean Bandit/Jess Glynne
4. 'Real Love' – Clean Bandit/Jess Glynne
5. 'Shotgun' – George Ezra
6. 'This Is Me' – Keala Settle
7. 'Haven't Met You Yet' – Michael Bublé
8. 'How Far I'll Go' – Auli'i Cravalho
9. 'She's So Lovely' – Scouting for Girls
10. 'All About You' – McFly

THE FAMILY'S FAVOURITE SONGS

1.

_____

2.

_____

3.

_____

4.

_____

5.

_____

6.

_____

7.

_____

8.

_____

9.

_____

10.

_____

The Coat Flip Hack

It can be a challenge for little ones to put a coat on themselves and with toddlers it can be the catalyst for a morning tantrum. This cool trick that will have them putting on their own coat in no time.

Lay the open coat on the floor in front of them with the top or hooded part in front of their feet. Get them to put their arms into each of the sleeves and flip the coat over their head. They will be so amazed, and once they have mastered it they'll be able to do it so fast their friends will think it's a magic trick.

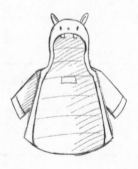

Two-Minute Teeth

Getting kids to brush their teeth can be a challenge, especially for two minutes, as that two minutes can seem like a lifetime. There are some great apps you can download for free that time two minutes, play fun songs and have characters dancing on screen. Some even reward you with stars or stickers once you've brushed your teeth for the correct amount of time so it feels more like a game than a chore. I've found since using these apps my kids will brush their teeth for much longer because they are motivated by the reward at the end. After a while it just becomes a habit as they automatically brush their teeth for longer.

Name It

Having a child at school and nursery means a lot of labelling. It's easy to start the year off well with everything neatly labelled, but by the end of the first term you have lost jumpers, drinks bottles and have absolutely no idea what happened to the P.E. kit. You can buy amazing name stickers online that label clothes, drinks bottles, pencils and everything else that your child takes to school. They last in the washer and dryer, and if you're putting them on drinks bottles that are dishwasher safe, they can go in there too. Now, if we need to get a new jumper, we can label it within seconds and it's easier to identify if it goes missing.

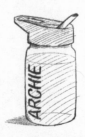

Dressing Gown

So you've got yourself ready for the day ahead and you're now sorting out the kids. A good way to stop your clean clothes getting covered in breakfast, sticky hands, snot or toothpaste, is to wear your dressing gown over your clothes. Take it off just before you leave the house and your clothes will avoid the morning wrath.

Evening
Hacks

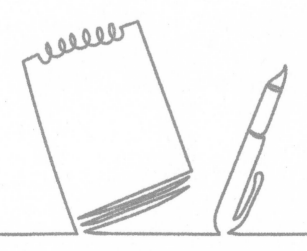

Depending on what stage you're at, your evenings as a mum might be the only time you get to relax and unwind, or you might be struggling to remember what an evening without feeding, winding and settling a baby looks like. I promise it gets easier eventually and you will be able to enjoy this time again! Before I sit down in the evenings there's a few things I like to make sure I've done to prepare for the next day.

Bedtime Routine

Try and keep the same routine every night. It can be difficult sometimes, but sticking to the same routine means that the kids know when it's bedtime and we don't have anyone fighting to stay up longer. After dinner, we let the boys stay up for about half an hour to an hour depending on what time we eat. Then we go up for a bath, read a book and go to bed.

I've found sticking to our evening routine as much as possible has really helped to avoid any tantrums about going to bed. Because they go up for a bath at the same time every night they know to expect it. Now our eldest is a bit older, we let him stay up a little longer to watch a movie on a Friday night and that really helps to break up the week and gives us something to look forward to.

To-Do List

Write your to-do list for the following day each evening. I think it really helps to get everything down on paper so you don't have it all in your head. Once you've written it down you can forget about it for the evening and get a good night's sleep before tackling it the next day.

Go to Bed Earlier

It often feels more of a challenge to get ourselves in a good bedtime routine than our children. Those hours between when the kids go to bed and when you do seem to fly by so it's easy for your bedtime to creep on, later and later. Try starting your bedtime routine fifteen minutes earlier each night so you gradually transition to having an earlier night. Even getting half an hour of extra sleep each night will help to improve your mood and wellbeing.

Preparation Is Key

It sounds obvious and a bit of a cliché, but getting everything you need for the next day ready the night before is one of my biggest tips. If you can have everyone's clothes laid out, bags ready and even the breakfast bowls and cereal boxes out ready and waiting it's amazing how much time it saves you each morning, and you'll be less stressed trying to run around doing it all.

Noted

If you're worried about forgetting something important – for example, if you're going on holiday and you need to remember important documents or you have to remember something for a meeting or school that day – leave a Post-it note on the front door the night before. That way, it will be the last thing you see before you leave the house and you can double-check you have it.

Keep It Clean

It can be really tempting to fall onto the sofa once you've conquered the kids' bedtime, but it's definitely worth making sure the house is clean before you relax for the evening, as once you sit down you won't feel like doing it. Simple things like making sure the dinner plates are cleaned or in the dishwasher, wiping down all the surfaces and putting the kids' toys away will help you enjoy your few hours of adult time and leave you with a clear head for the next day. Morning-you will definitely thank evening-you for getting it done.

Self-Care Hacks

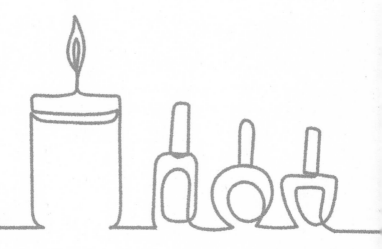

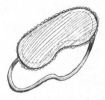

Make time for yourself every single day. We hear this so often and I guarantee the majority of us think it's impossible. With busy family lives, jobs or homes to clean, where can we possibly squeeze in any me time? But it's so important and vital for our mental health. How can we be expected to do it all and juggle so many tasks without feeling recharged and ready to tackle what we need to do? Have a look at your diary and usual routine and work out at which point of the day you could block out some time for you. It might be that some days you have longer to spend on yourself than others but even ten to fifteen minutes doing something that makes you happy can dramatically lift your mood. Whether it's a bubble bath with your favourite products after a long day, going for a run or doing some yoga to get your endorphins going, or meeting up with a friend for a coffee and a good chat, even the little things can make a difference. You can't pour from an empty cup, so fill it up with things you love and you'll find that you'll come back to your responsibilities better than ever.

I know it's hard to find the time for putting yourself first, so below I've started you off with thirty-one simple self-care activities that you can incorporate into your day. I like to think of this as a month-of-self-care challenge.

Day 1: Take a bubble bath

This is one of the best ways to relax and unwind after a long day. Find your favourite bath products – you know, those ones you save for special occasions – and use them. Light some scented candles and put on some music or your favourite movie or TV show on your phone or tablet and have a long soak.

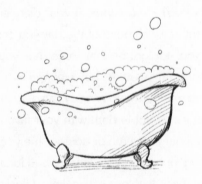

Day 2: Coffee with a friend

Talking is like therapy, so call or text a friend and arrange to meet up for a coffee. You can enjoy a break, put the world to rights and come back feeling refreshed. A problem shared is a problem halved so confide in someone close to you if you have things on your mind. I'm sure they will be more than happy that you chose to speak to them and you can get someone else's opinion which might clear your head and make things easier.

Day 3: Paint your nails

It's a simple one, but indulging in something that makes you feel like you've taken care of yourself will make you feel happier. Whether it's treating yourself to a proper manicure or doing it yourself at home, you can alternate between the two depending on time and budget. You could even have a go at doing your own gel nails at home with an LED nail lamp and polish.

Day 4: Do a YouTube yoga routine

If you don't feel like you have enough time to attend regular gym classes, why not do some at home? If you're a beginner, then you can search through thousands of online videos to find a routine or a course that's right for you. Yoga is a really gentle way to exercise and it's good for your mind, body and spirit. Start simple and work your way up. You can also do quick classes if you only have ten to fifteen minutes to spend on it.

Day 5: Go for a run

I feel as though it takes quite a lot of willpower to get out and run, especially if you're beginner – it can seem really daunting. However, it's one of the best forms of exercise and with some perseverance and practice you can build your endurance and actually begin to enjoy running.

Use apps like Couch to 5K to help you start at a slower pace and gradually run farther for longer each week until you've built up to 5K. As we know, endorphins make you happy! And once you've got into the habit, you're likely to feel happier and healthier.

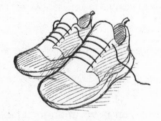

Day 6: Date night

Being parents can put a strain on any relationship and it's easy to forget what you were both like as a couple before kids. Call in a favour from your parents or a family member and see if they will babysit for you so you can go out for a drink and a nice meal and concentrate on your relationship for a couple of hours. Even though you'll probably spend most of the time talking about the kids, it gives you both a break and you'll remember why you fell in love in the first place.

Day 7: Call a loved one and have a long chat

If you've been meaning to call someone, but life just keeps getting in the way, set some time aside to ring them and have a long chat. I'm sure they will appreciate it and benefit from it just as much as you and you'll be glad you called them to talk.

Day 8: Light your favourite candles

Scents you enjoy can lift your mood. I love lighting certain candles according to the seasons: floral and fresh scents in the spring; fruity and ocean-based scents in the summer; warming, earthy scents in the autumn; and baking and festive scents in winter. Don't save your candles just because they look pretty – enjoy them through the seasons. I also love to burn candles full of essential oils, or add them to a diffuser, for a calming evening that gives your home a spa-like feel. Lavender is great for helping you relax, so keep an eye out for that scent.

Day 9: Get crafty!

Art can be really therapeutic, so raid the kids' art supplies once they've gone to bed. Practise some mindfulness in the form of drawing or painting. Take up crochet or embroidery and make something you can proudly display or give as a gift.

Day 10: Learn a new skill

You may feel like you've neglected yourself and your goals for a while. Let's face it, being a mum means sacrificing some things, at least for a while. Use your free time to learn a new skill that interests you. It could be cooking, photography or a new language – there are so many online tutorials and courses you can follow to learn a new skill and, you never know, it could turn into something you could make a new career out of or that could give you another income stream. Or just keep it as something you do to wind down in the evening whilst watching your favourite programme.

Day 11: Go to bed early

Sometimes all we need to feel a fresh sense of perspective is to go to bed earlier and have a good night's sleep. Instead of watching TV or looking at your phone before bed, you could try making sure you turn off all screens an hour before you go to sleep. The blue light of screens interferes with our body's natural ability to sleep, so reading a book can help you to relax and fall asleep faster.

Day 12: Write in a journal

Journalling can be as simple or creative as you like, a place to write down your thoughts at the end of the day and get them out of your head and onto paper. Journals can also be used to draw or write lists and there are again many YouTube videos to show you how to get creative with your journalling. If you love to write this could be a great way to relax.

Day 13: Tell yourself three things you love about yourself

Practise self-love by telling yourself three things you genuinely love about yourself. Something you've achieved or overcome in your life, a part of your body that you love or something that makes you feel happy and grateful. We often internally speak negatively to ourselves but this is a great way to turn that around and really look at the positive, amazing things about you.

We always see the worst in ourselves or berate ourselves for the things we perceive as failures, whether it is the way we look or feelings of guilt that we're not good enough parents. The truth is, when you look at yourself, these problems you see are magnified 100 times more than how anyone else sees or thinks of you. For example, I really struggle to leave the house without make-up. It stems from many years of having acne as a teenager and in my twenties and being left with a lot of scarring. The result is that I have never felt comfortable without a layer of foundation on my face and I feel like if I went outside with my natural skin everyone would be staring at me. As I've gotten older, though, I've started to notice that not everyone has perfect skin either, it's what makes us different and unique, and no one cares about it half as much as I do. Whatever your hang-ups, find ways to be confident in your skin. Something as simple as popping to the shops without make-up on really helps to boost my confidence and ability to go out to other places *au naturel*. We need to look in the mirror and see the positives – your body has done something incredible by growing and birthing a baby! And your scars and your stretch marks tell your story.

Day 14: Enjoy a meal with your partner once the kids have gone to bed

Even though going out for a date night is something lovely to look forward to, it's not always easy to get a babysitter, so an evening at home with a takeaway, a glass of wine and a movie can be just as special, plus the bonus is you can wear your pyjamas if you want to! It's still a great way to reconnect with your partner and enjoy some time together without worrying about the stresses of daily life.

Day 15: Go for a walk

Sometimes when it feels like you're spinning too many plates and you just need to get some headspace, a good walk is what you need – either with family, friends or on your own to give you time to think. You can then come back and focus on what you need to do with a clearer head.

Day 16: Watch your favourite movie

Self-care can sometimes be as simple as putting on your favourite movie, grabbing a few snacks and curling up under a cosy blanket. I love lots of different movie genres, everything from thrillers, to comedies, to chick flicks, and I have to be in the right mood to watch a certain film. But when it comes to self-care and relaxing, there are certain movies that I know will instantly feel like a big hug and give me that cosy feeling. Here are some of my favourites:

Movies to Make You Feel Cosy
1. *About Time*
2. *Father of the Bride 1 & 2*
3. *How to Lose a Guy in 10 Days*
4. *The Devil Wears Prada*
5. *You've Got Mail*

6. *Hook*
7. *Pretty Woman*
8. *Notting Hill*
9. *The Holiday*
10. *Mamma Mia*

Movies to Make You Cry

1. *A Walk to Remember*
2. *A Star Is Born*
3. *Marley and Me*
4. *My Girl*
5. *Stepmom*
6. *Moulin Rouge*
7. *Up*
8. *Forrest Gump*
9. *The Lion King*
10. Never Let Me Go

Movies to Make You Laugh

1. *Knocked Up*
2. *Bridesmaids*
3. *The Hangover*
4. *Meet the Parents*
5. *Mrs Doubtfire*

6. *Game Night*
7. *Shaun of the Dead*
8. *Bridget Jones's Diary*
9. *The Wedding Singer*
10. *We're the Millers*

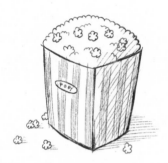

Day 17: Practise gratitude

It's easy to concentrate on the things we don't have in life rather than what we do. It's good to have goals and dreams, but finding the balance and practising gratitude for the things you already do have helps to keep you balanced and allows you to enjoy life without always chasing what you want next. Write a list of all of the things you're grateful for, so you can always see how far you've come and what you've achieved.

Day 18: Buy yourself flowers, or buy some seeds to grow your own

Treat yourself to a beautiful bunch of flowers – who says you have to have them bought for you? I love the way flowers instantly bring life to a space. If you want to do something that's more time-consuming but more satisfying in the long run, why don't you plant your own flowers from seeds and watch them grow. You can take pride in the fact that you've grown something yourself and for next to no money.

Day 19: Read a book

Reading is a fantastic way to distract your brain and transport you into a different world for a while. When you need a break from reality and the stresses of everyday life having a book to escape into can be a wonderful thing. It's also much better than scrolling through your phone or watching TV before you go to sleep.

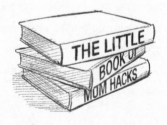

Day 20: Organise a space

Organising something in your space, whether it be a huge clean and declutter in your bedroom or tackling a messy drawer, can really help to focus your mind. Completing a task also allows you to feel proud of something you've achieved and enjoy your space more. If everything has a place to go then it's always going to be easy to put things away, so focus on finding a home for everything and don't be afraid to donate or sell things if you no longer have room for them or feel they work in your home.

Day 21: Dance to your favourite music

Put on a playlist that makes you feel happy, energetic, positive, calm, tranquil – whatever mood you're in, there's a playlist for it and if you're feeling happy, then those happy tunes are going to amplify that. Why not try listening to how you're feeling and if you know that your current mindset is negative or unhappy, listen to music that will have the opposite effect.

Music can completely change your mood. So when you need to shift gears and get out of a rut, listen to some music that will balance how you're feeling. If you're feeling on edge, a soothing and relaxing playlist might help you to calm down. If you need to get motivated but you're feeling a bit lethargic, put on something that will lift your mood and get the cogs in your brain turning. We have greater access to music now than ever before and there are some amazing streaming apps that have ready-made playlists for every mood. So next time you're feeling out of sorts, play some positive tunes and watch your mood turn around.

Day 22: Create a vision board

If you ever feel a bit lost and aren't quite sure how to achieve your goals and dreams, vision boarding is a great way to see the things you want in front of you and makes them more real and achievable. Start by thinking about what you want for your life and things you would like to achieve in the next five years. Then you can scour the internet for images that depict those dreams. You create your vision board by copy and pasting images to a photo editing app, adding them to a Pinterest board or printing them out and sticking them onto paper – whatever you choose to do, it's easier to see the full vision when it's all pulled together in front of you. It's a really powerful way to help manifest your dreams.

Day 23: Listen to a motivational podcast

Listening to an inspiring, motivational podcast can sometimes be just what you need if you're feeling a bit down and unpro-ductive. This really helps me to get back on track and remember what my goals are and what I want to achieve. Put one on whilst doing some organising or cleaning and it might even help you get the job done faster. My favourite podcasts for mums and parents include:

1. *Happy Mum, Happy Baby* – Giovanna Fletcher
2. *Mothers' Meeting with Lousie Pentland* – Louise Pentland (I was very honoured to be a guest on one episode!)
3. *Here We Go Again* – Stacey Solomon
4. *Sh**ged Married Annoyed* – Chris and Rosie Ramsey

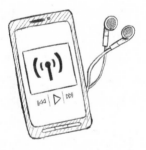

Day 24: Do something you used to love but don't get to do as much any more

If you had a hobby or passion that you used to love and devote a lot of time to, but life and commitments have got in the way, why not try and set some time aside to do it again. It could be a sport, creative activity, a style of dance, anything that used to make you happy and feel positive. It could be that you only manage to do one class or spend an hour on it a week, but even that's better than not doing it at all. Starting up a once-loved hobby after a long time can be really scary and intimidating, so see if a friend wants to join you so you don't feel quite so vulnerable, and remember, you don't need to put so much pressure on it because it's meant to be for fun.

Day 25: Unplug from social media

This might come as a surprise tip from me, seeing as my job is social media, but I really think it's important to have time away from your phone. Many of us are addicted to technology and can find ourselves constantly and mindlessly scrolling through apps and before we know it it's gone from something we downloaded for fun, that we check every now and again or to share a couple of photos, to obsessing and comparing ourselves to other people and their lives. There have been many times when I've found social media affects my mental health, as often you feel your life is lacking something that you see others with right in front of your eyes. Don't get me wrong, I have found social media wonderful for so many things. It's amazing for finding like-minded people, getting inspiration for your home or your wardrobe, not to mention I've made some amazing friends through our joint love of the app. But I feel as the social media giants grow, and the algorithm becomes smarter, it constantly finds new ways to keep you scrolling and posting for longer.

For this reason, I find it really important to set myself times when I don't go on my socials. I've mentioned earlier trying not to look at it before the school run and picking up my phone and laptop from after 9 a.m. like I would if I were working in an office. It's definitely something I'm working on, and I find it really hard to stay off it, as it's a big part of my job, but it's all about finding a balance. And if you're going through something in your life where seeing certain posts or topics upsets or triggers you, it's a good time to have a clear-out of people's content that you either don't enjoy any more or is making you feel anything less than happy and inspired. If you don't want to simply delete people, you can also mute content for a time and see how you feel after a while of not seeing their posts any more. It's simple to do and the other person won't even see that you've muted them.

Day 26: Put on a face mask
No, I'm not talking about the face-covering kind. Give your skin a pamper with a nourishing face mask. Depending on what your skin is lacking, use a mask to help brighten, smooth or make your skin glow like a goddess. You could even give a DIY mask a try.

Day 27: Learn about something new that interests you

Is there something that's always interested in you, but you've never really taken the time to learn more about it? Why not start researching the subject and learn something new. Take a course or read a book about it.

Day 28: Tidy your desktop

Whether you take that to mean the one you sit at to work or the one on your computer, chances are it needs a bit of an organise. Much like organising a space in our homes, organising our work environment or computer can really help to clear our minds and keep us focused on the project we're working on.

I often find myself with hundreds of icons all over my desktop and I can never find anything. But whenever I clean it up and put everything in its proper folder, I feel so much more productive and get things done quicker.

If you work from a desk, it's also a good time to go through the drawers and the clutter that builds up on top of your desk and get rid of paperwork or items you no longer need to stream-line your space.

Day 29: Take a nap

I know I've spoken a lot about getting motivated, achieving

dreams and reaching our goals, but it's good to know when to stop as well. We work so hard trying to make every aspect of our life perfect and, in reality, it's just not possible. Can you imagine a baby or toddler ever feeling guilty for taking a nap? No, because they need it, they need to rest in order to function, and even though of course as adults it's not necessary to take a nap, sometimes it helps to hit the reset button and realise that the world won't stop if you do for a little while. Learn to listen to your body and mind and take breaks when you need to.

Day 30: Read some inspiring quotes

Quotes can be very powerful. Sometimes we just need to read something that we connect with at the right moment to feel like we can deal with a situation that might have seemed too much for us to handle. Often it's that we can't quite find the words to explain how we're feeling and we don't have the belief in our-selves to make positive changes. Choose a few favourite quotes and keep them on your phone or printed out on your mirror or fridge to read them when you need a confidence boost and more motivation.

Day 31: Go to the movies

If all else fails, go to the movies! It's a great way to zone out of real life for an hour or two with no distractions, and concentrate on something completely different.

FAVOURITE SELF-CARE PRODUCTS

Self-care is not selfish and sometimes it's nice to spend a little money on something that will make you feel a lot better. Here are some of my favourite things to treat myself to when I need a pick-me-up:

HAIR WRAPS

I love putting my hair in a microfibre hair wrap after I've washed it. It's so much lighter than wrapping a towel around your head and it stays in place with a little loop and button on the back. Leaving your hair to dry for longer means you'll use less heat when it comes to drying it off.

BATH TRAY

I don't feel like my bath is complete without a bath tray containing everything I need within easy reach: my bubbles, a drink, some chocolate, and a good book or TV show on my phone, to name a few! They are so handy and make the experience seem so much more luxurious.

WEIGHTED BLANKET

Weighted blankets mimic a technique called Deep Touch Pressure therapy and can help to calm anxiety, reduce pain and improve your mood, as they can help you get a better night's sleep. They come in different weights to suit different people – for example, a child would need a lighter blanket than an adult.

ESSENTIAL-OIL DIFFUSER

You can use essential oils to improve your mood. Fill the diffuser with water and a few drops of your favourite essential oils to release a beautiful aroma into the air. They're also a great alternative to candles as you're only using a few drops of oil each time, so you get a lot of uses out of one bottle. I personally love to add lavender to mine to help me feel calm and relaxed.

SILK PILLOWCASE

This is a gorgeous luxury which, while more expensive than your average pillowcase, actually has added benefits for your hair and skin. Not only does it feel super opulent to lay your head on silk when it's time to sleep, but because the fibres have a smoother surface than cotton, they can help reduce wrinkles and keep frizzy hair at bay as there is less friction on your face and hair as you're moving around in the night.

JOURNAL

As I talked about it in the self-care hacks above, I had to mention a journal as one of my self-care must-haves. Writing can be very therapeutic and become a real hobby. Plus, they're a great keepsake to look back on years later.

BATH BOMBS

I really love a bath bomb! There's just something so satisfying about watching it fizz away and then jumping into a colourful bath of silky soft water. I like to throw one in the bath every now and then so it feels like a real treat!

PILLOW SPRAY

A calming pillow spray is something I've enjoyed using for years now. I like to think of it as the final step in my bedtime routine and the scents of lavender and chamomile always help me drift off to sleep.

BATH PILLOW

Talking of pillows, once you try a bath pillow, you'll never know how you lived without one. As you can probably tell, I do love a luxurious bath as the ultimate way to give myself some self-care. So adding an inflatable bath pillow into the mix is a game changer. If you haven't already tried one give it a go.

COSY SOCKS

A cosy pair of socks and a hot cup of tea on a cold day is one of life's simplest pleasures, and sometimes, self-care is as simple as finding the joy in the simple things.

No Heat Curls

A final handy tip that I wanted to share: you can use a dressing gown rope to curl your hair. It takes a little bit of practice but once you get it right it really works and leaves long-lasting curls with little effort. I find that it works best on dry hair, or after I have rough dried it.

Divide your hair into two sections. Lay the dressing gown rope over the top of your head and start by wrapping a front section of your hair around the rope away from your head. Then join that up with a piece from the back and continue wrapping it round, picking up another section from the front then the back as you go. At the end wrap any remaining hair around the rope and tie with a hair band. Do the same on the other side. Then you can just leave it loose or gently tie it behind your head in a soft scrunchie.

Travel Hacks

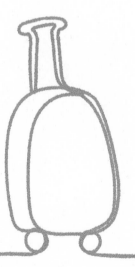

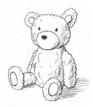

Getting the chance to travel, whether it's a road trip for a day at the beach or a flight to a bucket-list destination, is one of the most incredible opportunities we get in life. The chance to create memories in new places is priceless, but the travelling part can often be stressful for everyone involved. We have been lucky enough to travel more in recent years, something that I didn't do often when I was younger, so it has been a steep learning curve for me and I've had to find new ways to make the experience enjoyable for us all. There have definitely been a few occasions where I've found myself standing in a queue in a boiling hot airport at 3 a.m. with one child who suddenly has the energy of an Olympic athlete doing laps around the baggage carousel and another who is in serious need of sleep, but has decided a better idea would be to scream as loud as possible instead. In these moments, I have often wondered 'Is this worth it?' But, after a good night's sleep and some breakfast in the sunshine, the answer is always yes, and once we're home, I forget about the tough parts and am itching to book somewhere else!

Spending a long time sitting in one place, stopping for regular toilet breaks and being out of the usual routine can be challenging, so here are some hacks for all ages and eventualities.

Road Trip Snack Box

Be prepared for the inevitable cries of 'I'm hungry' on long road trips. Pack your child a road trip snack box, which will mean you don't have to make quite so many stops. Try using a box with lots of different compartments and fill them with different foods, such as pretzels, dried fruit, nuts, crackers and any of their favourite snacks. If your road trip is fairly short, you could include some chopped fruits and vegetables and even turn one of the compartments into a dip holder filled with houmous for a healthier option.

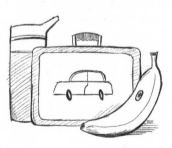

Portable Changing Station

Having a changing station in the back of your car is super handy in case you get caught out by forgetting your changing bag or running out of nappies whilst you're on the road. Keep a well-stocked box of nappies, wipes, nappy cream, nappy bags and a change of clothes as well as a travel changing mat in the boot of the car, so you're prepared for all eventualities.

DIY Car Air Freshener

A great way to create your own car air freshener that's cheap and natural is to simply take a wooden peg, cover it in five to ten drops of your favourite essential oil and attach it to the air vents in your car. You can do this in a few different places and the air will help the scent circulate around the car. You can top them up with more drops of oil as needed, or for a longer-lasting effect, take a hot glue gun and stick a few pom poms or a piece of felt to the peg. Adding the oils to the fabric will hold on to the scent even longer.

Travel Bin

It's all too easy for empty wrappers, bottles and paper to quickly fill up your car footwells on a road trip. To combat this, make a simple travel bin to keep your car spotless.

Just take an empty plastic cereal container, line it with a bag and cover it with the lid. Then you can easily open it up, fill with rubbish and close the lid, so if it falls over after going over any bumps, the rubbish stays inside. You can then empty it out at your next stop.

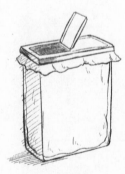

Caddies

Caddies with suction cups are great for sticking on your kid's car windows to help keep their things organised and within close reach. They could have a few stuck to their window with small toys, snacks or games inside that you want to be easily accessible for them. You can usually find them in discount or pound shops, often in the bathroom section.

WHAT TO PACK IN YOUR
CARRY-ON BAG

Since we started travelling on planes with our kids, plane bags have been a real winner. We fill them up with things to keep the kids entertained on the flight and it's something they now really look forward to and has become a little start to the holiday tradition. You can make them up according to the age of your child, but some of the best things we've packed are:

- Stickers
- Colouring books
- Pens on a string, or colour-magic pens and books that only apply colour to the paper, with no risk of them drawing all over the plane
- Small surprise toys

- Old toys they haven't seen for a while
- A tablet and headphones with their favourite games and a few movies or TV shows
- Playing cards or other card games such as Dobble and Top Trumps
- Story books
- Cosy pyjamas to change into for night flights
- Brain training toys such as a Rubik's Cube
- Favourite soft toy

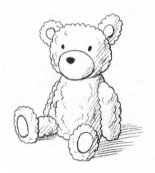

Plane Snacks

You may wonder why snacks weren't included on the previous list, but we learnt very quickly that giving the kids free rein over when they ate their snacks meant that they were gone very quickly and by the middle of the flight they were asking for more. We now like to keep all of the snacks in our bags and drip feed them throughout the flight, so they are spread out. We do give them a few sweet treats such as lollipops for when we're taking off and landing, but we also learnt that too many sweets and all the sugar resulted in hyper children and that's not what you need on a flight where you want them to be as well behaved as possible.

Don't Forget the Journey Home!

A rookie mistake is to forget that you also have to get through the journey home, which can sometimes be more stressful than the flight there, as everyone is out of routine and a bit deflated that the holiday is nearly over. So, don't forget to divide things up and keep a few items back for the way home. Some things can be repacked, such as pens and games, but save specific items, such as toys that they didn't play with on the way there, a fresh pair of pyjamas and of course the same amount of snacks that you needed for the first flight.

Multitasking Teddy

The right kind of teddy can be an excellent addition to pack in a kid's carry-on bag. As well as giving your child comfort, it can also double as a neck pillow for nap time or a night flight and if you put it on the tray in front of your child, you can prop your phone or tablet up on its feet to create a stand. Test some out at home before you leave to see which one works best.

Make Luggage Recognisable

If your luggage is quite a common style or colour, tie some fabric that's brightly coloured or with a recognisable pattern to your suitcase handles. This will save so much time when you're waiting for the bags to come round on the conveyor belt as you will spot it straight away.

Baby Powder

If you're heading to the beach on your trip, pack a small bottle of baby powder in your beach bag. It helps to quickly remove wet sand as the baby powder absorbs moisture, so after a quick pat down you'll be sand-free. This is especially helpful if you have kids that don't like the feeling of sand being stuck to them.

Hide Your Valuables

Whilst at the beach or around the pool, hide your valuables in something that a potential thief wouldn't think to take. For example, you can wrap your phone, wallet and other valuables up in a clean nappy and keep it inside your bag. Just make sure everyone in the family knows not to throw it away! You could also keep small valuable items in an empty sun cream bottle at the bottom of your bag.

Celebration
Hacks

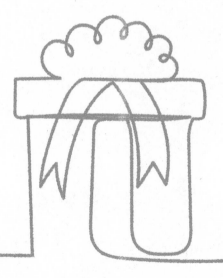

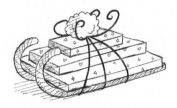

We all look forward to special occasions and celebrating with loved ones. They're a chance to get together, make memories and mark milestones. But sometimes the preparation for big events such as birthdays and Christmas can feel a little overwhelming. There have been a few occasions where we left things to the last minute. The evening before my son's third birthday we were out buying some last-minute presents and got stuck in three hours of traffic! We still had the presents to wrap, decorations to put up and my husband was adamant that he wanted to make the birthday cake from scratch. Needless to say, we were up until 2 a.m. and we definitely learnt our lesson to be more organised! Here are some ideas to make the planning and prep simpler and less stressful.

Digital Invites

Gone are the days when you had to handwrite each invite and wait for RSVPs to return. Now you can create a digital invite instead and send it to all of the guests in one click. Apps such as Evite allow you to easily create a digital invite and email or text it instead. Guests can then RSVP with the click of a button and you will have a list of everyone that is able to make it. Plus, it's better for the environment!

If you're still a fan of sending a paper invite though, you can create your own with apps such as Canva. It gives you templates to get started, and you can enter all of the information to save you having to write it out twenty-five times. Simply print them out at home and include your number so that people can RSVP.

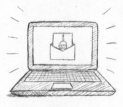

Who's It From?

If you've ever had a birthday party for your child, you'll know that it can be difficult to keep track of which presents came from which child to be able to thank them. Next time your child goes to a birthday party, stick the card to the actual present and then wrap it up so that when they unwrap it the card is inside and there's no confusion about who the present is from. It's also a good idea to have a pen and paper with you whilst your child unwraps any presents after a party so that you can thank individual people for their gifts. (That's if you can keep up with them!)

Stay Chilled

Instead of putting ice in your alcoholic drinks, add in frozen grapes or berries so you don't dilute the drink. If you want to make a child-friendly version, you could infuse water with their favourite frozen fruits to add flavour and keep drinks cool in a healthy and colourful way.

Smart Snacks

To make a quick 'Chip n Dip' bowl when entertaining, take a large bowl and put a wine glass in the middle. Then fill the bowl with crisps and the wine glass with a dip and place on the table. You could make it child-friendly by swapping in some carrots and cucumber sticks with dips that children are likely to love, such as sour cream or houmous.

Cheers!

If you're serving drinks for guests and you don't want to keep going back and forth to the kitchen, grab a muffin tin and use it as a makeshift drinks tray to easily serve everyone at the same time and keep the drinks more secure than a tray.

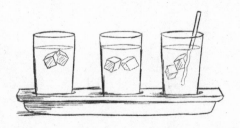

Wrap It Up

It's always difficult to know where to store wrapping paper. Why not hide it away in a suit bag and hang it on the back of a cupboard door or inside your wardrobe. It keeps all of your wrapping paper organised and together and you always know where it is when you need to wrap a present.

Sweet Treats

Make your own candy cane sleighs full of treats. These are so simple to make but kids and adults alike love them. Take two candy canes with the hooked ends facing up. Place three or four chocolate bars on top of them starting with the largest and most square to create a sleigh shape. You can even add on a bag of chocolate coins to look like Santa's sack and a small Santa-shaped chocolate on the front. Tie with some ribbon to keep it all together and finish the look.

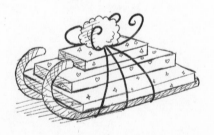

Hot Chocolate

Making gifts for loved ones is more time consuming but it can mean so much more when it's something handmade, personalised or thoughtful. If you're trying to save a bit of money why not make up some hot chocolate gift sets with the kids for the chocoholics in your life. Take a jar and fill it with the ingredients on the next page. You can attach a little note explaining how the recipient makes the hot chocolate, but they should be able to get around four to six hot chocolate drinks out of the mixture.

Hot Chocolate Recipe

You Will Need:

A jar

A gift tag

A piece of twine or string to attach the gift tag

¼ cup unsweetened cocoa powder

2 tablespoons sugar

¼ cup chocolate chips

Marshmallows to fill the rest of the jar

Depending on what flavour you want to make you could also add in some toffee chips, dark chocolate, crushed up candy canes, or even make a white chocolate version

* * *

If you're having people over for a festive gathering, there is nothing better than a little hot chocolate station set up in the kitchen. The recipe on the following page is perfect as it uses a slow cooker, which means you can put it on early and focus on other things ahead of the party. To be honest, this makes my mouth water just thinking about it. Plus the children will love decorating their own drinks for a special treat.

Slow cooker hot chocolate

You Will Need:

Slow cooker

1 litre of milk

250ml of double cream

300g of chocolate (we like milk chocolate but you can mix a few different ones or choose your favourite kind)

Marshmallows, squirty cream, candy canes, chocolate sprinkles or any other toppings you and your child might like (you can also add Irish cream for an adult-only version!)

Method:

Pour the milk and double cream into the slow cooker. Then break up the chocolate into small pieces and stir into the liquid. Leave to cook on low for 2 hours.

When your guests arrive they can help themselves or you can ladle it into cups and let them add all the toppings they would like. If you're having people over for a festive gathering, there is nothing better than a little hot chocolate station set up in the kitchen. To be honest, this makes my mouth water just thinking about it. Plus the children will love decorating their own drinks for a special treat.

Scrapbooks

Creating scrapbooks for your family to look back on is a great way to document special occasions. You can make them with your kids as a fun family activity, turning it into a tradition, and it means that all your photos don't just sit in your phone but become tangible and something you can share when friends and family come around.

An instant camera or printer is a great way to get photos off your phone and onto the page. You could also glue on ticket stubs, maps or leaflets if you went somewhere for the day, things you found along the way, such as a lucky penny or a leaf from a walk, and write about what you did. As your children get older they can contribute to writing in it as well and you could also add in things like a copy of their Christmas lists or letters to Santa from that year or drawings they do. It will become such a special keepsake to look back on over the years.

Open When . . .

A lovely gift idea is to create a set of envelopes for someone special to open at certain times. Some examples are 'Open when you need cheering up' and inside would be a page of jokes you know that person would like. 'Open when you miss me' could include lots of reasons why you love the person. 'Open when you need a treat' could include a gift voucher or gift card to the cinema. All you really need are some envelopes and some pens to decorate them, so it's very cost-effective and a gift that could really mean a lot, but of course you could add in treats to make it as extravagant as you want too.

It would also be a lovely way to show your children how much you care. As a mum, it's so special to receive a note or drawing from our children, but we don't always think how lovely it would be for them to receive one back. You could even do a version of this as a homemade advent calendar, with a little note every day alongside or instead of a chocolate to make it more meaningful.

Christmas Scene

If you have a large flat-based vase or hurricane jar, instead of filling it with flowers or candles you can create your very own Winter Wonderland Christmas scene inside. It makes a great activity for the whole family and, if you want, you can each work on your own one and create a story when they all come together!

Fill the bottom with flour to create the look of snow, and then add little figurines or small festive ornaments such as bottle-brush trees to make a woodland scene. I usually find Christmas

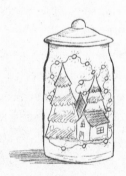

tree decorations work really well for this, as they're small and you should be able to find everything you need to create a festive scene such as Santa figures, houses, reindeer, presents and fairy lights. You just cut off the ribbon and add it in – you may even be able to repurpose some old decorations that have broken. The kids love making them and they're a beautiful piece to display on a shelf over Christmas. A bit like a snow globe except you definitely don't want to shake this one!

Twinkling Jars

You can also use similar vases and hurricane jars to create more glamorous-looking Christmas decorations. Take a string of battery-operated fairy lights and start adding them to the bottom of the jar, then add in some baubles that match your colour scheme, and continue to add the lights and more baubles until the jar is full. When you turn on the lights they will give off a beautiful glow. Remember to keep the battery pack near the top of the vase so you don't have to keep reaching in to turn it on and off.

Ribbon Roll

Use a kitchen roll holder to neatly store reels of ribbon. Ribbon can get really tangled and messy and that's not what you need when you have mountains of presents to wrap and not a lot of time. So storing the reels of ribbon on a kitchen roll holder is a great way to keep it organised and to see what you have easily. You can then just pull and cut bits off as needed.

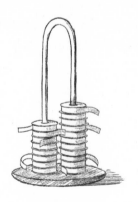

Tree Fragrance

Use fragrance sticks to scent your artificial tree. You can find these in most garden centres and DIY stores around Christmas time. They come in a few different scents – use pine if you want your tree to smell like the real thing or buy berry- or orange-scented ones to fragrance your house with a cosy, warming smell.

If you want to make some yourself and go down the more traditional route, you could add some cinnamon sticks, dried orange slices or clove-studded oranges to your tree. Your home will be smelling beautiful all season long.

Brown Paper Packages

Make your own wrapping paper with some simple brown paper and paint. You can splatter white paint onto it to create the look of snow. All you need to do is lay the paper out on some plastic sheets, lightly cover a clean toothbrush in white paint and flick it onto the paper; it doesn't take very long and creates a pretty effect. The kids also love to get involved so you can make it into an activity for the whole family. Use stencils or stamps or even handwrite someone's name or initial onto the presents to make it personalised. Finally, tie the presents up with twine for a rustic look or any colourful ribbon to match your theme.

If you don't feel like decorating the paper, why not just add a few finishing touches instead with some ribbon, twine and sprigs of fresh eucalyptus or rosemary, or look for an artificial sprig of mistletoe or berries – you'll find that you can get loads of present embellishments out of one sprig.

Eggcellent

Recycle your old egg cartons by using them as Christmas decoration storage. Each time you use up a box of eggs through the year, put them to one side (or store them in the loft) and when it comes to taking your decorations down after Christmas you'll have the perfect storage for some of your smaller or precious decorations. You could also store large baubles and ornaments in paper cups. Add the empty cups to a deep storage box; once you've filled them all up, lay some cardboard across the top and start a new layer. Stack them until the box is full, and your decorations will be safe and organised until next year.

Re-use Christmas Cards

Keep hold of your old Christmas cards and turn them into next year's gift tags. This works especially well for small cards with nice images on the front, or larger cards that have individual pictures on that you can cut out. If your child is old enough to use scissors, help them cut the front of the card off and use the other side to write the person's name and greeting.

Find the Gherkin

A fun idea for a family tradition is to buy a quirky Christmas tree ornament. The more unusual the better. Each year you can hide it in the tree and the first person to find it wins a prize. It sounds so simple but this is the sort of thing your children will remember as one of the best parts of Christmas and they may even carry on the tradition with their own children one day!

A little note from me

I was thinking about how I could sum this book up. It has been such a rewarding and fun experience getting to write it. One that was a little scary at times with the pressure to make it the best it could possibly be, or frustrating at points when I couldn't find the right words, but something that I feel so privileged to have been given the opportunity and responsibility to do and would do it all over again in a heartbeat, and then it hit me: that is exactly how I would sum up my experience so far of being a mum! So, I guess I can call this my book baby. Thank you so much for taking the time to read it. I hope it's given you some inspiration and some clever ideas to share with your mum friends or even pass on to your own children one day. I'd love to hear what you thought of it! You can find me on Instagram @katebow-bow and on my YouTube channel, Kate Murnane!

Lots of Love

Kate x

Acknowledgements

With the risk of sounding like I'm accepting an Oscar, I would love to take the opportunity to thank a few people. Firstly, my children Archie and Elliot. You made me a mum, you changed my entire life and made me happier than I ever knew I could be. And to my amazing husband Rikki. Meeting at school at seventeen, the odds were probably against us, but we've made such an amazing life for ourselves since those days and everything paid off in the end. Thank you for being the most supportive, patient person I know and being the ying to my yang.

Mum and Dad, my heroes. You have always been there for me and show me what unconditional love is. It isn't until you become a parent yourself you truly realise the effort and sacrifices your own parents made. And my brother, my partner in crime, you're either a comedian or my life coach, there is no in between. My wonderful grandparents. You inspire me every day and I feel so blessed to have you. You fill my life with sunshine.

My management team, Channel Mum, who work so hard behind the scenes and support me with my ideas and ambitions. And a big thank you to my editor Ru and the team at Orion Publishing Group for giving me the opportunity to write this book and achieve something that was always on my bucket list!

And finally, a big thank you to you for reading this book. Whether you bought it because you have been with me since my first video ten years ago, found me through my pregnancy and baby journey or simply picked up the book for some friendly tips and advice from a fellow mum, thank you, because I wouldn't have got to do this without you.

About the author

Kate Murnane is a much-loved lifestyle and mum YouTuber and influencer with over 488k followers across her social platforms and over thirty million views on YouTube. She was named in the *Mother & Baby* Mum List 2020 and lives in Kent with her husband and two boys. *The Little Book of Mum Hacks* is her first book.